John England

Blood Gases

The Basics – And A Little More

Table of Contents

Disclaimer..4

Preface..5

Introduction..7

1: Blood Gas Reports...9

2: Interpretation..13

3: Report Contents..14

4: How To Read A Blood Gas Report....................................20

5: Respiratory Acidosis...28

6: Respiratory Alkalosis..40

7: Metabolic Alkalosis...50

8: Metabolic Acidosis..60

9: Case Study...81

10: Self Test...86

11: Self Test Answers..91

Appendix 1: Glossary..94

Appendix 2: Arterial Blood Gas Assay................................124

Appendix 3: Acid-Base Balance...125

Appendix 4: Mixed Acid-Base Conditions..........................126

Appendix 5: Expected Compensation..................................127

Appendix 6: Oxygen-Hb Dissociation...128

Appendix 7: pH -> paCO2..129

Appendix 8: Anion Gap..130

Books By John England..132

Disclaimer

The author has made every effort to ensure that the contents of this book are correct, error free, and a reasonable representation of the design goal, which is to introduce the reader to the process of analysing blood gas assays (reports), with particular focus on oxygenation and acid-base balance disturbances.

The author accepts no responsibility or liability for damages caused by any erroneous contents of this book and, in all situations, recommends that professional guidelines, national policies, and direction from suitably qualified medical staff take precedence over the information contained herein.

All rights reserved. The contents of this book may not be duplicated or distributed in any form, without written permission from the author.

√ √ √ √ √ √

Preface

The effective delivery of healthcare is determined by providing patients with treatments that are appropriate to their conditions, and those treatments are, themselves, determined by accurate diagnosis of those ill-health conditions. A blood gas report, or assay, is one of a suite of facilities that help the physician to understand the patient's health disturbances, and the underlying causes of those disturbances, particularly with patients who are subject to critical care.

Nurses and allied staff, such as anaesthetic technicians (ATs) and operating department practitioners (ODPs), must also be able to recognise, at least to a basic level, blood gas reports, although not to the same level as physicians, such as anaesthetists and intensivists (Note: for brevity, future references to nurses also includes ATs and ODPs.)

This book has been specifically designed to introduce nurses to a step-by-step method of blood gas analysis, that includes a tabular technique that gives graphical clues about what primary and compensatory mechanisms the patient is experiencing. The aim is to instil the reader with a systematic way of "reading" blood gas reports, without the distraction of discussing issues of pathology, pharmacology, or pathophysiology. The emphasis, throughout, is method, not medical.

After reading this book, the reader will have gained competence in one

Preface

of the most useful and important diagnostic techniques available to critical care staff, and will have increased their ability to understand and anticipate the patient's changing condition.

Being able to read blood gases, incidentally, is also quite satisfying, and definitely raises the profile and professionalism of any nurse who has that ability.

√ √ √ √ √ √ √

Introduction

Blood Gases introduces the reader to the process of analysing a blood gas report, with the primary aim of identifying problems or irregularities with oxygenation and acid-base balance. Clinical and pathophysiological issues have been, in the main, excluded from the content, because this book concerns itself with technicalities and methods of blood gas analysis, rather than with the medical, legal, or professional matters that are part of the scope of critical patient care.

The text has been broken down into easily digestible chapters and, as much as possible, the main content has been limited to the most essential details of blood gas analysis, with the more technical aspects extracted to the Appendices. In this way, the reader can choose to focus solely on the fundamental aspects of blood gas analysis, and leave the slightly more complex issues for study at a later time.

The first four chapters introduce the theory of blood gases, describe the main components of a blood gas report, and present a step-by-step method of discerning what the individual and collective values mean, with respect to the patient's condition, and the possible reasons for abnormal report values.

Chapters five to eight give examples of the four types of primary acid-base disturbance, with the chapter on metabolic acidosis given special

Introduction

focus, because of the particular techniques of acid-base analysis that are available for deciphering the types and causes of a metabolic acidosis.

The final two chapters comprise a self test and answers, which the user is expected to tackle with reference to the four acid-base chapters.

There then follows the Appendices, including a Glossary of terms and principles, which is for the interested reader, but not essential for anyone who just wants to concentrate on the basic technique of reading a blood gas report.

√ √ √ √ √ √

1: Blood Gas Reports

The effective delivery of healthcare is dependent on the identification of a patient's "dis-ease", finding the causes for relevant conditions, and taking remedial action to mitigate the causes to reverse the disease processes. To find the causes of a patient's medical problem, a variety of standard techniques are used to distinguish between the different signs and processes that the patient might be suffering from. Those techniques include observations, clinical history, patient/carer evidence, monitoring, biopsies, and analyses of blood and urine, which includes interpretation of blood gases.

Utility

Blood gas values shows how well a patient is ventilating, and how well oxygenated the blood is. Similar information is given on how well the body is removing carbon dioxide, and balancing acid and base levels, which helps illustrate the function of the lungs, liver, and kidneys. Values for particular electrolytes show how well homeostatic mechanisms are performing, and can give warning to imbalances that might deteriorate; lactate (metabolite) levels can reveal problems such as anaerobic respiration, and whether or not sepsis might be developing; glucose values can reveal ketone build-up, which is particularly important in sufferers of diabetes mellitus, and a sequence of blood gas reports uncovers trends and patterns in the patient's changing condition.

The Blood Gas Assay

A blood sample is fed into a blood gas machine, and a report is produced that lists values for: pH, gases (dissolved oxygen [pO_2] and carbon dioxide [pCO_2] pressures, bicarbonate), oximetry (Hb, O_2 saturation), electrolytes (sodium, potassium, chloride, calcium), and metabolites (glucose, lactate, bilirubin), haematocrit, and albumin. The blood sample can be taken from a vein, artery, or capillary (infants), and there is very little difference between the different sources, except that only arterial blood (ABG) gives an accurate state of dissolved oxygen and carbon dioxide. The disadvantage of taking an arterial sample is that, unless an arterial line is in place, it is very painful for the patient, so should be avoided, unless ventilation (O_2, CO_2) information is needed, such as with critical care and major surgical patients. In this text, we assume that blood samples are taken from arterial lines.

Blood Samples

A blood sample must be taken properly, so that no errors are introduced into the analysis process. To that end, blood sampling protocols must be followed or, in their absence, gas machine manufacturer guidelines. Some general rules, for arterial lines, include ensuring the blood gas machine is within service date, an appropriate and in-date heparanised blood gas syringe is used, the sample is taken after arterial line saline solution has been aspirated, does not contain air bubbles, the syringe is gently rolled in the hand, but not agitated, and is taken to the blood gas machine for analysis without delay.

Limitations

A blood gas report gives a lot of useful information to attending doctors, particularly anaesthetists. Knowledgeable nurses, especially those in Critical and Intensive Care Units, also benefit from such information, because it helps them understand and monitor patterns of change, and reveals how effective treatments are. However, by itself, a blood gas report may not reveal all information revealing the causes of any physiological imbalance, so the report should be used in conjunction with other investigations, such as the patient's clinical record, comprehensive blood and urine reports, and standard monitored parameters. This holistic approach helps support or refute any suppositions that the attending clinicians may form, and supporting information might be required before definitive diagnostic conclusions are made.

As useful as a blood gas report is, it should always be used within the context of a larger comprehensive diagnostic scheme, and consideration should be given to underlying patient problems, such as COPD, which can hide a state of normality for the patient, with values that are abnormal for other patients. An example of this is where a COPD patient's "normal" (chronic) HCO_3 (bicarbonate) is, say, 33 mmol/L, with high CO_2 and pH, making it appear that the patient has developed a part compensated metabolic alkalosis when, in fact, these values may be ongoing baseline values, and normal for the patient, who is hyperventilating due to low arterial oxygen pressure (respiratory failure). Such a complication is beyond the scope of this text, where the emphasis is on learning the basic rules of acid-base interpretation.

Nurse Ability

The ability to interpret a blood gas report, and gain greater insight into what is happening to the patient, helps the nurse act as a "check" for the actions of a doctor who, like any other person, can make mistakes in interpretation and treatment decisions. By spotting errors, the nurse, inevitably, reduces risk to the patient, and those nurses who do make the effort to raise their blood gas interpretation skills, always stand out as being superior professionals, who are well thought of by doctors and colleagues. The learning process, though, for understanding blood gases may be lengthy, but is well worth the effort and, once mastered, it is a very satisfying skill to have. Anyone can do it – it just takes persistence.

√ √ √ √ √ √ √

2: Interpretation

The exact format and entries for a blood gas report can be different for different models of blood gas machine, and particular setups, but the principle entries are common to all machines, and the main ones are discussed in this book, as listed in Appendix 2.

Summary descriptions of the various entries are itemised in the Glossary (Appendix 1), but it is not necessary to have more than a basic familiarity with the different report entries in order to be able to decipher either the oxygenation or acid-base irregularities necessary for blood gas interpretation.

For completeness, some discussions of essential science concepts are repeated throughout, but a lack of understanding of some of those matters of basic science does not prevent being able to successfully analyse a blood gas report, so do not worry if the chemistry etc. is unknown to you.

√ √ √ √ √ √ √

3: Report Contents

General Principles

Blood gas reports contain most of the basic information with which to decipher oxygenation and acid-base conditions, but not all of the entries are needed for development of blood gas interpretation skills, making some of them redundant for initial learning purposes, so they will be generally excluded, or only included in specific contexts of discussion. Example entries that will be excluded (mostly) from discussion are haematocrit, albumin, Base Excess, and bilirubin. By reducing the "clutter" of these and other entries, important as they are, the reader can more easily focus on developing the skill in blood gas interpretation - these other entries can be studied at leisure.

When referring to blood gas values, such as oxygen partial pressure, it is far easier to use symbolic notation which, in this case, is pO_2, rather than write out the full "oxygen partial pressure", so this is the format used in this text. Additionally, if the source of the pO_2 is arterial, there is no need to write out "arterial", instead, "a" is included in the prefix, forming "paO_2"; if the source is venous, "pvO_2" is used, and "pcO_2" for capillary blood. Note, however, blood gas machines do not print these source letters – they simply use the core symbol, such as "pO_2".

Therefore, we will follow this convention, which is fine, because we know the source of the blood - arterial – because we took it!

Please also note also that blood gas machines may report pressure values in kiloPascals (kPa) or millimetres of mercury (mmHg), so it is essential to be able to convert between these two measurement systems. As the pascal is an S.I. derived unit, it is the preferred pressure system, but staff have to comply with local protocols, so there may not always be much choice in which to use. This should not be a problem, however, because converting from kPa to mmHg is just a matter of multiplying by 7.5, and dividing mmHg by 7.5 to convert to kPa. In this text, both units are used, and with mmHg for compensation calculations.

The following descriptions are supplementary to those in the Glossary, where there are more detailed descriptions.

Entries

Albumin

The most abundant plasma protein and unmeasured anion, which serves to maintain osmotic pressure, nourishes tissues, carries hormones and drugs, and stops blood from leaking into the extravascular space. A reduced level (due to nephrotic syndrome, liver problems, shock, or inflammation) causes increased chloride, so can make a high anion gap metabolic acidosis (HAGMA) appear like a normal anion gap metabolic acidosis (NAGMA); a 1 gram drop in albumin decreases anion gap by 2-3 mmol, so accurate albumin measurement is essential to avoid "finding" the wrong reason for the acidosis. Note: dehydration increases albumin levels.

Cl-

Chlorine ion, and the main anion in the Anion Gap calculation. Range: 95-108 mmol/litre.

Glucose

A sugar molecule that is necessary for normal aerobic metabolism. A low level can lead to anaerobic metabolism, ketone build up, and ketoacidosis. Range: 3.6 - 5.3 mmol/litre.

Haematocrit (Hct)

The fractional volume of blood occupied by red blood cells. Low levels cause hypoxia. An apparent high level might be a low level disguised by dehydration. Normal range: 0.4-0.5 (men), and 0.37–0.45 (women).

Haemoglobin (Hb)

Transports oxygen. Normal range of arterial haemoglobin is 140 to 180 g/litre for men, and 120 to 160 g/litre for women. A low Hb count might be due to iron deficiency, anaemia, cancer, vitamin deficiency, hypothyroidism, pregnancy, urinary infection, or liver disease.

HCO_3-

Bicarbonate: a buffer to donate H+ ions in the alkalotic patient, and mop up H+ ions in acidotic conditions. Normal range is 22-26 mmol/litre. Lower than 22 indicates an acidosis, and above 26 is alkalosis. Used in conjunction with pH and pCO_2 to determine if an acidosis/alkalosis is of a primary respiratory or metabolic nature, or if it is compensation for such. Part of the *Bicarbonate Buffer Equation*.

K+
Cation of potassium. Also part of the Anion Gap calculation, although often omitted. Range: 3.5-5.3 mmol/litre.

Lactate
An electrolyte marker for anaerobic (no oxygen) metabolism, and often an indicator of sepsis. Lactic acidosis occurs when lactate is > 4, and is of 2 types: A and B (see Glossary). Range: 0.5 - 1.6 mmol/litre.

Na+
Cation of sodium. Na+ is one of the electrolytes used in the Anion Gap calculation, which helps to determine causes of metabolic acidosis. Range: 133-146 mmol/litre.

pCO_2
Partial pressure of carbon dioxide, with normal range being 4.7–6 kPa (35-45 mmHg). If pCO_2 is low (hypocapnia), the usual cause is hyperventilation, which blows off H+ ions, thereby allowing an alkalotic condition to develop. A high value (hypercapnia) is the opposite case – hypoventilation allows CO_2 to be retained, causing an acidosis. If a change in pCO_2 is a compensatory reaction to a metabolic acid-base imbalance, it might take several hours before full or final compensation is reached, perhaps even as long as 24 hours. Contrast that with the 1-5 days it takes for a metabolic compensation for a respiratory acid-base imbalance to occur - a respiratory compensation is relatively quick.

pH
Blood pH values above 7, but below 7.4, are classed as acidic, and above

7.4 are alkali. Above 7.45 is alkalaemia, and below 7.35 is acidaemia.

The measured pH value is either normal (7.4), or it has been changed by bodily respiratory or metabolic processes, which have to be discerned by reviewing other values, such as CO_2, HCO_3-, minute volume, clinical and drug records, and so on. Collectively, these other parameters can help reveal what acid-base imbalance processes are in progress, and what compensatory mechanisms may be in play. What this means is that pH shows the particular acid-base condition of the blood but not, by itself, what acidotic or alkalotic processes are happening – these have to be worked out from CO_2, bicarbonate (HCO_3-), and Anion Gap.

pO2

The three entries that most describe how well a patient is being oxygenated are pO_2 (partial pressure of oxygen), sometimes referred to as *oxygen tension*), SO_2 (% oxygen saturation), and Hb (haemoglobin) count. If pO_2 is low, there may not be sufficient pressure gradient for oxygen to diffuse to the tissues, resulting in hypoxia. The cause of the low pO_2 must be found and addressed without delay, and immediate steps may include giving supplemental oxygen, sitting the patient up (increases FRC), or ensuring there is no disruption to O_2 supply, such as disconnection, airway obstruction, laryngospasm, bronchospasm, and so on. Naturally, the degree of urgency is dependent on the pO_2 value, and the attending nurse or doctor should never hesitate in calling for help when the patient is not receiving an adequate supply of oxygen, because that will, inevitably, quickly proceed to an emergency situation, and where intubation might be necessary.

A normal value for pO_2 is 10 kPa less than FiO_2 (Fraction of Inspired oxygen), so, if breathing room air (assume 101 kPa, 760 mmHg), FiO_2 (minus water vapour) is approximately 20%, so pO_2 should be 10-13.3

kPa (75-100 mmHg). A pO$_2$ below 10 kPa means hypoxaemia and, if pO$_2$ falls below 8 kPa (mmHg), it is classed as respiratory failure, and an emergency.

If the patient is intubated and breathing, for example, an FiO$_2$ of 30%, the expected pO$_2$ will be ~ 20 kPa (150 mmHg). In this case, if pO$_2$ is less than the expected 20 kPa, there may be sufficient oxygen tension to feed the patient's tissues, but there may be a problem of oxygen supply, which might be a problem of ventilation (V) or perfusion (Q), which must, invariably, be reported to the responsible clinician, such as an anaesthetist, and immediately investigated.

SO$_2$

% of haemoglobin (Hb) saturated with oxygen; a healthy range is 95-100%, but a low value might be normal for a COPD patient. If SO$_2$ is low, but pO$_2$ is normal, the cause might be defective Hb, or carbon monoxide poisoning, so these should be considered with the overall oxygenation status. It must be remembered that the reliability of an SO$_2$ value is dependant on how the value is found; if the blood gas machine actually measures the value, rather than calculates it, the SO$_2$ must differentiate between Hb bound with oxygen, and Hb that might be bound with carbon monoxide, so the SO$_2$ value is probably reliable.

However, if the value is derived from pO$_2$, using an internal look-up table (Appendix 6) which, itself, is based on the Oxygen-Hb Dissociation Curve, the value may only be accurate if there are no defective Hb molecules, and if none of the Hb is bound with carbon monoxide. Remember that if SO$_2$ is 100%, but there is only, say, 80% of the normal count of Hb molecules, a truer SO$_2$ will be 80%, not 100%.

√ √ √ √ √ √ √

4: How To Read A Blood Gas Report

A blood gas report can be described as containing three main groups of information for: oxygenation, acid-base balance, and values for specific components (electrolytes, glucose etc). Because the primary function of the respiratory and circulatory systems is to deliver oxygen to the tissues, it makes sense to prioritise assessment of the oxygenation over the other factors, so that will be the format followed in this book – oxygenation first!

Note that it is essential to develop the ability to refer to the various report entries by their commonly used biological names and chemical symbols, rather than writing out their full names, because that is how clinicians communicate with each other. For example, when making initial references to bicarbonate, "bicarbonate" is written out, then followed with "HCO_3^-" in parenthesis, because it leaves no possibility of confusion, in case a similar chemical symbol is included in the text. But, after the first few occasions that it is written in full, references to bicarbonate (or any other entity/particle) should be made by its chemical symbol, "HCO_3^-".

Using symbols is a real time saver, and is the way that chemical information is communicated on blood gas reports. Note: reference ranges for the various blood gas entries are given in Appendix 2. Note also that "~" reads as "approximately".

Oxygenation

Firstly, work out what a normal value for pO_2 should be, based on the FiO_2, as described in the previous chapter. If the patient is breathing room air, pO_2 should be ~10-13.3 kPa (75-100 mmHg) but, if pO_2 is significantly low, it should be reported and corrected, otherwise it should be monitored to see if it is stable, or deteriorating. The value for SO_2 should also be considered in oxygenation: does it correspond with the pO_2 value (Appendix 6), or is it lower than expected?

If SO_2 is at an acceptable level, are you certain it is reliable, for the reasons described in the previous chapter (measured or calculated)? Could the SO_2 value be corrupted by carbon monoxide content? Is there a possibility of a low red blood cell count (haematocrit), and is there normal Hb to carry an adequate level of oxygen to the tissues? Also, is the patient anaemic, and how could it be degrading oxygenation?

Priority is oxygenation and, because ventilation can collapse into hypoxia in an instant, ventilation and tissue oxygenation must be continuously monitored, rapidly assessed, and immediately managed.

Acid-base Balance

The list of common acid-base disturbances and combinations are listed in Appendix 3, with normal values listed in Appendix 2, and it is worth making note of these, to use as a guide for working out the examples given in the chapters on blood gas analysis.

The objectives of understanding acid-base imbalance are threefold: **Firstly**, what is the pH of the blood? **Secondly**, what primary respiratory or metabolic processes and compensations are causing that particularly pH level? **Thirdly**, what is causing those processes? Once the underlying causes of the imbalances are found, treatment options can be considered and implemented.

Regardless of what the pH is, the values for HCO_3^- and pCO_2 must be looked at as well as the pH, even if pH is 7.4 (normal), because those values will reveal why the pH value is what it is, and whether or not a normal or abnormal pH is due to primary and compensatory acidotic/alkalotic mechanisms.

So, for example, if pH is lower than 7.4, the question to ask is "What is causing this acidotic state?". If it is a failure of the respiratory system to expire a level of CO_2 that matches the amount of CO_2 the body is producing, then the acidity is due to hypoventilation and CO_2 being retained. Alternatively, if the reason for the acidity is not of a respiratory nature, it must be due to excess acid production, reduced excretion of $H+$ ions, a drop in the level of HCO_3^- (bicarbonate), or some trauma or genetic problem.

In some cases, a particular imbalance might be anticipated, perhaps because the patient has a known kidney dysfunction that prevents normal excretion of $H+$, or addition of new bicarbonate, so some of the blood gas readings might be predictable.

It is one of the advantages, for nurses, who understand blood gas reports, that they are able to anticipate both what acid-base disturbances the patient has, or will develop, and what equipment and drugs might be needed to correct those imbalances. Often, of course, a nurse will know from experience that acid-base management will be needed for certain patients, such as diabetes mellitus sufferers, and those with pulmonary or renal dysfunction. Experience has value.

Once the type of imbalance is found (respiratory or metabolic, acidic or alkalotic), interventions have to be decided, and these can be as simple as addressing the hyperventilation of an anxious patient, or stimulating the breathing of a hypoventilating patient. For more complicated metabolic conditions, the reasons why there is too much or too little of something have to be found, and that might be something that seems not directly connected with acid-base problems; infection, for example, might be having a negative affect on tissue oxygenation, or a low potassium (hypokalaemia) level might be affecting cardiac output, thereby leading to a perfusion problem, and so resulting in anaerobic metabolism, and consequent increased lactate acidity.

For the nurse, who does not have the experience to be aware of these clinical issues, duty is best served by simply understanding that something is not right, and bringing that to the attention of the responsible physician. Nurses must be able to identify that something is wrong, and what the general cause of the problem is (metabolic alkalosis etc), but they don't necessarily have to understand the medical situation – that is the doctor's job.

Imbalances

An acid-base imbalance can be one of four types, with two being of a respiratory nature, and two metabolic:

* Respiratory Acidosis – pH is below 7.35, and pCO_2 is above the normal (mean) value of 5.3 kPa (40 mmHg).

* Respiratory Alkalosis - pH is above 7.45, and pCO_2 is below the normal value of 5.3 kPa (40 mmHg).

* Metabolic Acidosis - pH is below 7.35, and HCO_3^- is below the normal value of 24 mmol/litre.

* Metabolic Alkalosis - pH is above 7.45, and HCO_3^- is above the normal value of 24 mmol/litre.

These conditions are described in the following chapters, but the essential attributes that describe each of the four imbalances should be memorised before continuing, because they provide the foundation, and first lesson, in learning acid-base disturbances.

Compensation

Formulae to calculate CO_2 or HCO_3^- compensation are given in Appendix 5.

Whenever pH differs from the "normal" value of 7.4, there is an acid-base imbalance, however small, that will usually trigger an automatic compensation by the complimentary system to the one causing the imbalance. For example, if there is a primary acidosis (caused by the respiratory system), due to excess pCO_2 retention, the body will naturally try to counter the acidosis with a response that attempts to raise pH to the normal range, and it does this by metabolic means which, specifically, means the kidneys expelling H+ ions, and raising the levels of the bicarbonate (HCO_3^-) buffer. If enough time has elapsed for full compensation to occur, pH will be pulled back up into the normal range of 7.35-7.45 (full compensation), unless there is another primary acidosis occurring (respiratory and metabolic acidoses), in which case it is a mixed disturbance, described later.

If compensation is occurring, but has not yet moved pH into the normal range, it is termed "partial compensation". Similar processes occur for the other three acid-base disturbances, and they will be made clear in later chapters.

Acute Vs Chronic Disturbances

As a general guide, if compensatory mechanisms have adjusted pH into the normal range (7.35-7.45) then the acid-base disturbance is

4: How To Read A Blood Gas Report

probably of a chronic nature. Otherwise, the disturbance is acute.

Graphical Representation

The table in Appendix 3 is a useful learning tool for learning the different combinations for acid-base imbalances. Similarly, another graphical system, taught in medical schools, can be used for plotting characteristics for particular cases; for example, an **uncompensated respiratory acidosis** (pH=7.2, HCO3-=26 mmol/L, pCO2=56 mmHg) would be tabulated as:

Low	*Normal*	*High*
pH	HCO3-	pCO2

My own version of the above tabular system adds two columns, which allow entries for values that are in their normal range, but either side of the mean value, as illustrated by tabulating the above respiratory acidosis as:

Low	Low range	Normal	High range	High
pH 7.2 (acid)			HCO3-, 26 mmol	pCO2 56 mmHg, 7.4 kPa

The difference is that, where the 3 column table indicates **uncompensated** respiratory acidosis, the 5 column method shows that there may, indeed, be a compensation developing, making this a border-line **partially compensated** respiratory acidosis. Also, by adding the values, it obviates the need to keep referring to the values elsewhere (*the addition of "Acid" or "Base" is not essential, but it does provide an extra prompt*). This tabular system will be repeated in the chapters containing worked examples, but it is not an essential part of acid-base interpretation – it is just a learning aid, so can be ignored, if preferred. Generally, though, this five column table system does give a helpful summary view of acid-base balance, and is a good starting point for progressing to more detailed analysis of any blood gas report.

Mixed Disturbances

The demarkation between those who have good blood gas interpretation skills, and others with more basic skills, concerns the ability to spot more than one primary acid base disturbance, as exemplified and summarised in Appendix 4. If the disturbances are opposing, where one is acidotic, and the other is alkalotic, similar to the way that compensation occurs, one disturbance will lower pH, and the other will raise it, and they may cancel out so that pH is brought into its normal range. In this way, it might appear that there is no acid-base disturbance at all, because pH is normal, when in fact there is both a respiratory and a metabolic disturbance in play.

Similarly, there may simultaneously be both a respiratory and metabolic disturbance, in which case the pH will be distinctly low (acidosis) or high (alkalosis), unless there is an effective compensation occurring, which will tend to push pH into the normal range (full compensation), or improved from its initial worst value (partial compensation). To make things interesting, three disturbances can occur simultaneously: metabolic acidosis and alkalosis, plus either respiratory acidosis or alkalosis - respiratory acidosis and respiratory alkalosis do NOT occur together. The skill is to spot the disturbances, and compensations, and identify the causes of each disturbance.

Other Values

Although discussion of clinical matters is beyond the scope of this book, it would be remit not to give brief mention to some of the other clinically significant entries listed on a blood gas report, because they are part and parcel of holistic diagnostics, so any abnormal values, such as for an electrolyte, for example, would require as much consideration for treatment as would acid-base disturbances.

For details of the following entries, refer to the Glossary (Appendix 1) and value reference (Appendix 2): Cl- (chloride), HCO_3^- (bicarbonate), K+ (potassium), Na+ (sodium), lactate, and glucose. With respect to acid-base balance, an appreciation of abnormal levels of lactate and glucose have special significance, because they are components of high Anion Gap metabolic acidosis (HAGMA), and identifying those abnormal levels is key to correcting the resultant acid-base imbalance. Sodium, potassium, chloride, and bicarbonate also have particular significance for acid-base analysis, because they allow determination of the type of a metabolic acidotic disturbance, through calculation of the afore-mentioned Anion Gap - discussed later.

Holistic Analysis

For emphasis, it is worth repeating that the blood gas report should not be relied upon independently. Instead, it should be used in conjunction with other information, observations, and assays, so that conclusions about causes and treatments are not determined by a single source – the blood gas report – but supported and reinforced by all available and relevant information.

√ √ √ √ √ √ √

5: Respiratory Acidosis

Respiratory acidosis is defined as the process that, unless compensated (kidneys), produces an acidotic state of the blood, which is a pH (see Glossary, Appendix 1) with a value lower than 7.4, and is usually due to hypoventilation, where under-breathing results in less CO_2 being breathed out than is being generated by the patient. Remember that true acidity only occurs when pH is lower than a value of 7, so anything above that is, strictly speaking, alkali but, as already mentioned, in the medical field, acidity is a relative term, and the "neutral" value is deemed to be 7.4, with acceptable tolerance +/- 0.05, giving a "normal" range of 7.35 – 7.45. If pH drops below 7.35, it is classed as an acidaemia, above 7.45 is an alkalaemia.

Once recognised, the cause of the respiratory acidosis must be found, so that it may be treated. Typical causes are: COPD, Myasthenia Gravis, Guillain-Barre Syndrome, and hypothyroidism.

For the intubated patient, resolution is often achieved by increasing minute volume; either through respiratory rate or tidal volume otherwise, for the attending nurse, recognition of the problem is paramount, so that the problem can be escalated to senior staff; diagnostic ability is a bonus, but is not the nurse's primary role.

Acute Respiratory Acidosis

Acute conditions can be due to several causes, although COPD and obesity are more likely to be causes in chronic cases, but there is no definite delineation of causes between acute and chronic cases. In acute cases, and before metabolic compensation with bicarbonate buffering takes place, initial buffering of H+ is intracellular, and achieved by haemoglobin and phosphate, so calculating early buffering with bicarbonate may not be so reliable but, for exercise purposes, just assume we are dealing with renal compensation with bicarbonate, using the calculation (see also Appendix 5) for expected HCO_3^- as:

$$24 + [\mathbf{0.1} * (\text{measured } pCO_2 - 40 \text{ mmHg})] \text{ mmol/litre} +/- 3$$

The resultant value can be a good guide and indication of whether the acidosis is acute or chronic, but is not an absolute indicator. Indeed, if there is a mixed case of two or more acid-base imbalances, the HCO_3^- level might be either lower or higher than expected, so the calculated expected value must be considered in context of the patient's overall condition, and not as a pure sign.

Chronic Respiratory Acidosis

A notable difference between acute and chronic respiratory acidosis is that of the type of patient concerned. Chronic sufferers usually understand their conditions, and will have clinical histories that reveal underlying causes and effectiveness of treatments. A COPD patient, for example, is likely to be a regular receiver of services, and their condition will be relatively easy to understand. Similarly for patients with Obesity Hypoventilation Syndrome, who receive ongoing support and monitoring. Another difference is that many chronic patients have well managed and stable conditions, with prolonged reabsorption of bicarbonate to maintain pH. It is also worth noting that a chronic sufferer of respiratory acidosis can also be occasionally affected by an acute instance of respiratory acidosis – just to make things interesting!

HCO_3^- compensation, in chronic cases, is slightly different from acute ones, and is given as:

$$HCO_3^- = 24 + \{\mathbf{0.4} * (\text{measured } pCO_2 - 40 \text{ mmHg})\} \text{ mmol/L}$$

COPD

Giving supplementary oxygen to COPD patients can be not so straight forward, due to them having a hypoxic rather than a respiratory drive. This should be documented and well understood by all nurses tending to the patient, otherwise a nurse might mistakenly use their initiative and make the **wrong decision** about supplementary oxygen.

Another thing to be cautious of, is the administration of sodium bicarbonate to acidotic patients, because it can cause a rapid swing in pH to an alkalotic state.

Blood Gas Examples

Examples are presented in a tabulated format, with components of the blood gas report discussed with respect to the oxygenation and acid-base situation. Please note that emphasis is on using a methodology to analyse blood gases, rather than considering clinical issues. To that end, only minimum report components are presented – missing values should be considered "normal" and, unless otherwise stated, assume enough time has passed for compensation to occur.

5: Respiratory Acidosis

Example 1

Entity	Value	Normal Range
pO2	9.2 kPa ↓ (69 mmHg), room air	10–13.3 kPa (75-100 mmHg)
SO2	93% ↓	95-100%
pH	7.2 ↓	7.35–7.45
pCO2	7.7 kPa ↑ (58 mmHg)	4.7–6 kPa (35-45 mmHg)
HCO3-	24 mmol/L	22-26 mmol/L

The patient, 28, admits to taking opiates, has hypotension, dry mouth, weakness, nausea, vision disturbance, and respiratory depression.

Oxygenation
Oxygen tension (9.2 kPa) and sats (93%) are slightly low, so this is mild hypoxaemia, apparently caused by drug induced respiratory depression.

Acid-Base
pH is below the normal range, showing an acute acidaemia.

Carbon Dioxide (pCO2)
CO2 is raised, so this is respiratory acidosis.

5: Respiratory Acidosis

Bicarbonate (HCO3-)

24 mmol/litre is normal, so no compensation seems to be occurring.

Acid-Base Table

Low	Low normal	Normal	High normal	High
pH 7.2 (acid)				
				pCO2 58 mmHg 7.7 kPa (acid)
		HCO3- 24 mmol	Expected HCO3- 26 mmol	

This table shows the advantage it has over the three column version, because it presents the pattern of an uncompensated respiratory acidosis, with just a glance. *Note: Adding "acid/alkali" is optional.*

Compensation

For **acute** respiratory acidosis, expected HCO3- compensation is:

$$HCO_3^- = 24 + [\mathbf{0.1} * (\text{measured pCO}_2 - 40 \text{ mmHg})]$$

$$24 + [0.1 * \mathbf{18}] = 26 \text{ mmol}$$

This is **respiratory acidosis without compensation.**

Example 2

Entity	Value	Normal Range
pO_2	8.2 kPa ↓ (62 mmHg), room air	10–13.3 kPa (75-100 mmHg)
SO_2	91% ↓	95-100%
pH	7.32 ↓	7.35–7.45
pCO_2	6.4 kPa ↑ (48 mmHg)	4.7–6 kPa (35-45 mmHg)
HCO_3^-	28 mmol/L ↑	22-26 mmol/L

Patient, 44, has tremors, is tired, sweating, and very anxious.

Oxygenation

O_2 tension (hypoxaemia) and sats are low, and close to hypoxic respiratory failure, so this is a case that could deteriorate quickly, and should be addressed promptly.

Acid-Base

The low pH, 7.32, means mild acidaemia.

Carbon Dioxide (pCO_2)

A CO_2 of 6.4 kPa (48 mmHg) is high and, if pO_2 falls below 8 kPa (60 mmHg), this will become hypercapnic respiratory failure (Type II).

Bicarbonate (HCO_3^-)

28 mmol/litre is above normal, and has been increased, by the kidneys, to buffer (mop up) excess H+ ions that cause the acidaemia.

Acid-Base Table

Low	Low normal	Normal	High normal	High
pH 7.32 (acid)				
				pCO_2 48 mmHg 6.4 kPa (acid)
			Expected HCO_3^- 25 mmol	HCO_3^- 28 mmol (alkali)

At a glance, this appears to be an acute primary respiratory acidosis with partial compensation.

Compensation

For **acute** respiratory acidosis, expected HCO_3^- compensation is:

$$HCO_3^- = 24 + [\mathbf{0.1} * (\text{measured } pCO_2 - 40 \text{ mmHg})],$$
$$24 + [\mathbf{0.1} * (48 - 40 \text{ mmHg})] = 25 \text{ mmol}$$

The expected 25 mmol is close to the measured 28 mmol. The pH is not yet in the normal range, making this a **respiratory acidosis with partial compensation** (Appendix 3, rule 4), which confirms what is indicated by the above acid-base table. Perhaps a few more hours will make compensation complete.

5: Respiratory Acidosis

Example 3

Entity	Value	Normal Range
pO2	9.8 kPa ↓ (74 mmHg), room air	10–13.3 kPa (75-100 mmHg)
SO2	94% ↓	95-100%
pH	7.35	7.35–7.45
pCO2	6.1 kPa (46 mmHg)	4.7–6 kPa (35-45 mmHg)
HCO3-	29 mmol/L ↑	22-26 mmol/L

Note: This example is similar to the previous example, but with a subtle difference - revealed by the acid-base table.

Oxygenation

O2 tension (hypoxaemia) and sats are at the lower margin of normal, so need close monitoring for deterioration.

Acid-Base

The pH 7.35 is slightly acidic, but in the normal range.

Carbon Dioxide (pCO2)

A CO2 of 6.1 kPa (46 mmHg) is high, pointing to respiratory acidosis, even though pH is normal.

Bicarbonate (HCO3-)

29 mmol/litre is above normal, and has been increased, by the kidneys,

5: Respiratory Acidosis

to buffer (mop up) excess H+ ions that cause the acidaemia.

Acid-Base Table

Low	Low normal	Normal	High normal	High
	pH 7.35 (acid)			
				pCO2 46 mmHg, 6.1 kPa (acid)
			Expected HCO3- 26 mmol	HCO3- 29 mmol (alkali)

The acid-base table graphically reveals that the primary imbalance is respiratory acidosis.

Compensation

For chronic respiratory acidosis (because it is compensated), expected HCO3- compensation is 24 + [**0.4** * (measured pCO2 − 40 mmHg)]:

$$HCO3^- = 24 + [\mathbf{0.4} * (46-40)] = 26 \text{ mmol}$$

The blood gas value of 29 mmol is within tolerance levels (26), so compensation appears as expected: this is **compensated respiratory acidosis** (Appendix 3, rule 4).

Example 4

Entity	Value	Normal Range
pO_2	7.6 kPa ↓ (57 mmHg), room air	10–13.3 kPa (75-100 mmHg)
SO_2	89% ↓	95-100%
pH	7.28 ↓	7.35–7.45
pCO_2	7.2 kPa ↑ (54 mmHg)	4.7–6 kPa (35-45 mmHg)
HCO_3^-	22 mmol/L	22-26 mmol/L

Oxygenation

Oxygen tension (pO_2) of 7.6 kPa and saturation (SO_2) of 89% indicate a ventilation or perfusion (V/Q) problem (probably hypoventilation), resulting in CO_2 retention, and pCO_2 shows that this is a Type II respiratory failure. This problem might possibly be something that is easily solved with supplementary oxygen, or addressing an obvious cause which, for an obese patient, might be something as simple as sitting them up, and giving them a little oxygen. However, until analysis from a physician is made, it should be considered a potential emergency, anaesthetic help should be called for, and the patient should be given supplemental oxygen, as an immediate intervention. If this is a deteriorating problem, CPAP, jet ventilation, or intubation may be necessary, so someone should be delegated to ensure these things are available. Note: calling for help from an anaesthetist or intensivist is ALWAYS recommended, even if a fellow nurse claims that the problem is minor, and not worth calling a doctor for (it does happen).

5: Respiratory Acidosis

In all cases, actions should be based on the best interests of the patient, including when it is not your patient who is experiencing whatever problem you observe. For emphasis: interfering in other cases may upset your colleagues but, if they don't have the necessary sense of urgency to advocate for patients, they are contravening safety protocols and, in particular, they are failing to comply with the Precautionary Principle – assume the worst, and act accordingly.

Acid-Base
pH 7.28 is acidaemia.

Carbon Dioxide (pCO2)
CO2 of 7.2 kPa 54 mmHg) is above normal, signifying respiratory acidosis. The patient is probably hypoventilating.

Bicarbonate (HCO3-)
HCO3- of 22 mmol is in the normal range, but borderline acidic.

Acid-Base Table

Low	Low normal	Normal	High normal	High
pH 7.28 (acid)				
				pCO2 54 mmHg, 7.2 kPa (acid)
	HCO3- 22 mmol		Expected HCO3- 25 mmol	

5: Respiratory Acidosis

The "at-a-glance" value of the table displays the typical pattern of a respiratory acidosis, with HCO3- also on the acidic side of normal.

Compensation

22 mmol is in the normal bicarbonate range, but on the acid side, so is evidence of little or no compensation for the respiratory acidosis, and gives a clue that this is an acute disturbance. Expected compensation in acute respiratory acidosis is given by:

$$HCO_3^- = 24 + [\mathbf{0.1} * (pCO_2 \text{ mmHg} - 40)] = 25.4 \text{ mmol}$$

The blood gas value of 22 mmol suggests that there may be a slight metabolic acidosis in addition to the respiratory acidosis.

Complication

With respect to acid-base balance, this is a **primary acute respiratory acidosis**, with a possible additional **primary metabolic acidosis** (Appendix 3, rule 5), although loss of bicarbonate (HCO3-) might possibly be due to diarrhoea or other GI losses.

The critical factor is oxygenation, and an arterial oxygen tension (pO2) of 7.6 kPa (57 mmHg) is **respiratory failure**. CO2 tension of 7.2 kPa (54 mmHg) is high, so the respiratory failure is **Type II** (hypercapnic), and this is the underlying cause of the acidaemia.

√ √ √ √ √ √ √

6: Respiratory Alkalosis

Respiratory alkalosis can occur when pH is above 7.4, and is defined as an alkalaemia, if pH is above 7.45; pCO$_2$ will be lower than 4.7 kPa (35 mmHg). Typically, the alkalosis is due to more CO$_2$ being expired (hyperventilation) than being produced, causing a reduced blood concentration of H+ ions, with resultant increase in pH. Pathological causes include: pulmonary embolism, sepsis, and aspirin overdose. If ventilated, reducing minute volume might lower pH.

Acute Respiratory Alkalosis
An acute respiratory alkalosis is usually differentiated from a chronic condition by little or no metabolic compensation. Typical causes of the hyperventilation are anxiety attacks, pain, pulmonary embolism, hypoxia, and pneumothorax. When enough time has elapsed long enough for some metabolic (kidneys) compensation to occur, the expected HCO$_3^-$ value is given by:

$$HCO_3^- = 24 - [\mathbf{0.2} * (40 - pCO_2\ mmHg)]\ mmol/litre$$

Chronic Respiratory Alkalosis
In chronic cases, metabolic compensation may bring pH to normal, or near normal, with expected HCO$_3^-$ calculated by:

$$HCO_3^- = 24 - [\mathbf{0.5} * (40 - pCO_2\ mmHg)]\ mmol/litre$$

Example 5

Entity	Value	Normal Range
pO_2	12.3 kPa (93 mmHg), room air	10–13.3 kPa (75-100 mmHg)
SO_2	97%	95-100%
pH	7.55 ↑	7.35–7.45
pCO_2	3.3 kPa ↓ (25 mmHg)	4.7–6 kPa (35-45 mmHg)
HCO_3^-	22 mmol/L	22-26 mmol/L

Oxygenation
Oxygen tension (pO_2) and saturation (SO_2) are normal.

Acid-Base
pH 7.55 is mildly alkalotic.

Carbon Dioxide (pCO_2)
CO_2 of 25 mmHg (3.3 kPa) is low, so this is a respiratory alkalosis. The patient is blowing off more CO_2 than the body is producing, which suggests hyperventilation.

Bicarbonate (HCO_3^-)
HCO_3^- of 22 is normal, but on the acidic side of the mean value of 24.

6: Respiratory Alkalosis

Acid-Base Table

Low	Low normal	Normal	High normal	High
				pH 7.55 (alkali)
pCO2 25 mmHg, 3.3 kPa (alkali)				
	HCO3- 22 mmol			

The table suggests respiratory alkalosis, with minimal or no compensation - an acute condition.

Compensation

Acute respiratory alkalosis expected compensation is:

$$HCO_3^- = 24 - [\mathbf{0.2} * (40 - pCO_2 \text{ mmHg})] = 21 \text{ mmol}$$

The HCO3- value of 22 mmol is close to what is expected. This appears to be a **partially compensated respiratory alkalosis** (Appendix 3, rule 9).

√ √ √ √ √ √ √

Example 6

Entity	Value	Normal Range
pO_2	29 kPa (218 mmHg)	30 kPa (40% FiO_2) (226 mmHg)
SO_2	99%	95-100%
pH	7.48 ↑	7.35–7.45
pCO_2	4.2 kPa ↓ (32 mmHg)	4.7–6 kPa (35-45 mmHg)
HCO_3^-	20 mmol/L ↓	22-26 mmol/L

Oxygenation

The patient is intubated, with a Fraction of Inspired Oxygen (FiO_2) set at 40%, so expected pO_2 is 30 kPa (226 mmHg). The blood gas pO_2 of 29 kPa (218 mmHg) is very close to what it should be for this FiO_2. Oxygen saturation (SO_2) is normal.

Acid-Base

pH of 7.48 is an alkalosis (alkalaemia).

Carbon Dioxide (pCO_2)

CO_2 of 32 mmHg (4.2 kPa) is below normal, and is consistent with respiratory alkalosis.

Bicarbonate (HCO_3^-)

HCO_3^- of 20 mmol is below (acidic side) the normal range, and is suggestive of metabolic compensation.

6: Respiratory Alkalosis

Acid-Base Table

Low	Low normal	Normal	High normal	High
				pH 7.48 (alkali)
pCO2 32 mmHg, 4.2 kPa (alkali)				
HCO3- 20 mmol (acid)				

The table provides an instant graphical reflection of partially compensated respiratory alkalosis.

Compensation

HCO3- (bicarbonate) compensation appears to be occurring (pH is near normal), and is signified by the expected HCO3- for chronic respiratory alkalosis, given by:

$$HCO_3^- = 24 - [\mathbf{0.5} * (40 - pCO_2 \text{ mmHg})] = 20 \text{ mmol}$$

which matches the ABG of 20 mmol. This is a **partially compensated acute respiratory alkalosis** (Appendix 3, rule 9).

√ √ √ √ √ √ √

Example 7

Entity	Value	Normal Range
pO2	27 kPa (203 mmHg)	30 kPa (**40% FiO2**) (226 mmHg)
SO2	99%	95-100%
pH	7.46 ↑	7.35–7.45
pCO2	3.8 kPa ↑ (28 mmHg)	4.7–6 kPa (35-45 mmHg)
HCO3-	12 mmol/L ↓	22-26 mmol/L

Note: this is a small variation of the previous example.

Oxygenation

The patient is intubated, with a Fraction of Inspired Oxygen (FiO2) set at 40%, so pO2 should be ~30 kPa (226 mmHg). The blood gas pO2 of 27 kPa (203 mmHg) is slightly less than the expected 30 kPa. Oxygen saturation (SO2) is normal.

Acid-Base

pH of 7.46 is a slight alkalosis (alkalaemia).

Carbon Dioxide (pCO2)

CO2 of 28 mmHg (3.8 kPa) is below normal (35 mmHg, 4.7 kPa), and is consistent with respiratory alkalosis.

6: Respiratory Alkalosis

Bicarbonate (HCO3-)

HCO3- of 12 mmol is well below (acidic side) the normal range, and is suggestive of metabolic compensation.

Acid-Base Table

Low	Low normal	Normal	High normal	High
				pH 7.46 (alkali)
pCO2 28 mmHg, 3.8 kPa (alkali)				
HCO3- 12 mmol (*Expected 18 mmol*)				

This appears to be a partially compensated respiratory alkalosis.

Compensation

HCO3- (bicarbonate) compensation is occurring, and is signified by the expected HCO3- for **chronic** respiratory alkalosis, given by:

$$HCO_3^- = 24 - [\mathbf{0.5} * (40 - pCO_2 \text{ mmHg})] = 18 \text{ mmol}$$

but is higher than the ABG value of 12 mmol, so the extra drop in HCO3- should be investigated: the bicarbonate loss due to e.g., diarrhoea, has produced an additional disturbance of a primary metabolic acidosis? Note how the HCO3- calculation has enabled the initial impression of a *compensated respiratory alkalosis* to be replaced by a more accurate **mixed respiratory alkalosis and metabolic acidosis**.

6: Respiratory Alkalosis

Example 8

Entity	Value	Normal Range
pO2	10.3 kPa (78 mmHg)	10–13.3 kPa (75-100 mmHg)
SO2	95%	95-100%
pH	7.6 ↑	7.35–7.45
pCO2	2.6 kPa ↓ (20 mmHg)	4.7–6 kPa (35-45 mmHg)
HCO3-	26 mmol/L	22-26 mmol/L

Oxygenation

The blood gas pO2 of 78 mmHg (10.3 kPa) and oxygen saturation (SO2) are normal - just.

Acid-Base

pH of 7.6 is an alkalosis (alkalaemia).

Carbon Dioxide (pCO2)

CO2 of 20 mmHg (2.6 kPa) is below normal, and is consistent with respiratory alkalosis (from over breathing).

Bicarbonate (HCO3-)

HCO3- of 26 mmol is at the top of the normal range, and is suggestive of a possible slight metabolic alkalosis.

6: Respiratory Alkalosis

Acid-Base Table

Low	Low normal	Normal	High normal	High
				pH 7.6 (alkali)
pCO2 20 mmHg, 2.6 kPa (alkali)				
	Expected HCO3- 20 mmol		HCO3- 26 mmol	

The table indicates respiratory alkalosis with a possible small additional metabolic alkalosis.

Compensation

If this is acute respiratory alkalosis, expected HCO3- compensation is:

$$HCO_3^- = 24 - [\mathbf{0.2} * (40 - pCO_2 \text{ mmHg})] = 20 \text{ mmol}$$

HCO3- of 20 and 14 mmol are both lower than the patient's 26 mmol – so this is a **mixed metabolic** and **respiratory alkalosis**.

√ √ √ √ √ √ √

7: Metabolic Alkalosis

Metabolic alkalosis is a process that can lead to an alkalaemia (pH > 7.45), with bicarbonate (HCO3-) greater than 26 mmol/L. The main reasons for metabolic alkalosis, are a loss of H+ ions (acid loss), typically due to vomiting, diuretics, or dehydration, or increased HCO3- in the blood (perhaps from too many antacids). Treatment might include potassium chloride (KCl). *{Tip: two clues for metabolic alkalosis are low potassium (K+) and chloride (Cl-) levels}*

Usually, respiratory compensation for metabolic alkalosis is by means of hypoventilation, and results in CO_2 retention, with consequent reduction in pH towards the normal range, commencing within an hour or so of the alkalosis starting. The increase in pCO_2 will be at a lower rate than the increase in bicarbonate, and any deviation from this rule can be an indication of an additional acid-base disturbance: increase in CO_2 more than expected (Appendix 5) might be due to a secondary disturbance of respiratory acidosis, whereas a smaller CO_2 increase could mean that the second disturbance is a respiratory alkalosis.

A check for the above additional disturbances is by means of the calculation of the expected CO_2 compensation:

$$pCO_2 = \mathbf{0.6 * (HCO_3^- - 24) + 40} \text{ mmHg}$$

Example 9

Entity	Value	Normal Range
pO_2	11.3 kPa (85 mmHg)	10–13.3 kPa (75-100 mmHg)
SO_2	96%	95-100%
pH	7.48 ↑	7.35–7.45
pCO_2	5.8 kPa (44 mmHg)	4.7–6 kPa (35-45 mmHg)
HCO_3^-	31 mmol/L ↑	22-26 mmol/L

Oxygenation
There is no apparent problem with oxygenation (assuming Hb and haematocrit are normal), for this patient who is breathing room air.

Acid-Base
pH of 7.48 means alkalaemia.

Carbon Dioxide (pCO_2)
CO_2 of 44 mmHg (5.8 kPa) is in the high part of the normal range, so there may be an alkalotic process occurring.

Bicarbonate (HCO_3^-)
HCO_3^- of 31 mmol is high and alkalotic, and corresponds with the pH, so this is a metabolic alkalosis.

7: Metabolic Alkalosis

Acid-Base Table

Low	Low normal	Normal	High normal	High
				pH 7.48 (alkali)
			pCO2 44 mmHg, 5.8 kPa	
				HCO3- 31 mmol (alkali)

The table confirms that this is an acute metabolic alkalosis.

Compensation

Expected respiratory carbon dioxide compensation is:

$$pCO_2 = \mathbf{0.6 * (HCO_3^- - 24) + 40} = 44 \text{ mmHg}$$

which exactly matches the blood gas value, so compensation is as expected for this **partially compensated metabolic alkalosis** (Appendix 3, rule 7).

√ √ √ √ √ √ √

Example 10

Entity	Value	Normal Range
pO2	12.4 kPa (97 mmHg)	10–13.3 kPa (75-100 mmHg)
SO2	98%	95-100%
pH	7.68 ↑	7.35–7.45
pCO2	4.9 kPa (37 mmHg)	4.7–6 kPa (35-45 mmHg)
HCO3-	40 mmol/L ↑	22-26 mmol/L
Cl-	80 mmol/L ↓	95-108 mmol/L

Oxygenation

O2 saturation (SO2) and partial pressure (pO2) are normal.

Acid-Base

pH of 7.68 is distinctly alkalotic.

Carbon Dioxide (pCO2)

CO2 of 37 mmHg (4.9 kPa) is on the low side of the normal range.

Bicarbonate (HCO3-)

HCO3- of 40 mmol is alkalotic and, because pH is also alkalotic, means there is a metabolic alkalosis present.

7: Metabolic Alkalosis

Acid-Base Table

Low	Low normal	Normal	High normal	High
				pH 7.68 (alkali)
	pCO2 37 mmHg, 4.9 kPa			Expected pCO2 50 mmHg
				HCO3- 40 mmol (alkali)

The values depict acute metabolic alkalosis, without compensation.

Compensation

Expected respiratory compensation is:

$$pCO_2 = \mathbf{0.6 * (HCO_3^- - 24) + 40} = 50 \text{ mmHg}$$

which is higher than the blood gas value of 37 mmHg, so respiratory compensation is lower than expected for a compensated metabolic alkalosis, which suggests there is an additional respiratory alkalosis occurring, making this a **mixed respiratory and metabolic alkalosis** (Appendix 3, rule 10).

Chloride (Cl-)

A low chloride level is an extra clue of a metabolic alkalosis.

√ √ √ √ √ √ √

Example 11

Entity	Value	Normal Range
pO2	8.4 kPa ↓ (63 mmHg)	10–13.3 kPa (75-100 mmHg)
SO2	91% ↓	95-100%
pH	7.46	7.35–7.45
pCO2	4.8 kPa ↓ (36 mmHg)	4.7–6 kPa (35-45 mmHg)
HCO3-	44 mmol/L ↑	22-26 mmol/L

Oxygenation

The low oxygen partial pressure is at the hypoxic level, and is only slightly higher than the value that describes respiratory failure - 8 kPa (60 mmHg). Together with the low saturation value (91%), this suggests this might be a patient who has significant chronic respiratory problems, such as COPD, in which case these values might be normal for him/her. Alternatively, there may be some more acute cause, such as drugs, CNS or chest injury, airway obstruction, ventilation or perfusion problems etc. No conclusion, therefore, can be drawn just from these oxygenation values alone, but the respiratory status must be addressed.

Acid-Base

With a hypoxic patient, it might be reasonable to expect that the patient's acid-base status would be on the acidic side, and with a pH lower than 7.35 but, with a given pH value of 7.46, this is not the case, because the pH is slightly alkalotic.

Carbon Dioxide (pCO2)

The pCO2 value of 4.8 kPa (36 mmHg) suggests hyperventilation. If so, the patient might be at risk of running out of energy for breathing, so, this is further evidence that their ventilation/perfusion status must be addressed.

Bicarbonate (HCO3-)

HCO3- of 44 mmol is alkalotic, and this ties in with the pH of 7.41, because it appears that, even though pH is in the normal range, rather than having the higher value that would be expected in an alkalotic disturbance, the pH has most probably been brought lower by a compensatory acidotic process of increased pCO2, which will be proved after calculating what the expected pCO2 should be, if it is, indeed, compensating for the alkalosis.

Acid-Base Table

Low	Low normal	Normal	High normal	High
			pH 7.41	
	pCO2 36 mmHg, 4.8 kPa (alkali)			Expected pCO2 52 mmHg, 6.9 kPa
				HCO3- 44 mmol (alkali)

The table displays the pattern for a chronic metabolic alkalosis, with pH and bicarbonate on the high side (right) of the table. However, for an expected respiratory compensation, the pCO2 value would also be on

7: Metabolic Alkalosis

the high side (see Appendix 3, rule 7) so, to cause the pCO2 to be on the low side, there must be an additional alkalotic process occurring, as listed in Appendix 3, rule 10.

Compensation

Expected respiratory compensation is:

$$pCO_2 = 0.6 * (HCO_3^- - 24) + 40 = 52 mmHg$$

but the patient's pCO2 is only 36 mmHg, so there must be an additional alkalotic (respiratory) process occurring, as deduced in the above "Acid-Base Table" section. This patient is experiencing a **mixed respiratory and metabolic alkalosis** (Appendix 3, rule 10).

√ √ √ √ √ √ √

Example 12

Entity	Value	Normal Range
pO2	12.1 kPa (97 mmHg)	10–13.3 kPa (75-100 mmHg)
SO2	96%	95-100%
pH	7.48 ↑	7.35–7.45
pCO2	5.3 kPa (40 mmHg)	4.7–6 kPa (35-45 mmHg)
HCO3-	27 mmol/L ↑	22-26 mmol/L

Oxygenation

Both pO2 and SO2 are normal.

Acid-Base

pH of 7.48 is slightly alkalotic.

Carbon Dioxide (pCO2)

CO2 of 40 mmHg (5.3 kPa) is perfectly normal.

Bicarbonate (HCO3-)

HCO3- of 27 mmol is just on the alkalotic side, and ties in with the pH of 7.48, which suggests metabolic alkalosis.

7: Metabolic Alkalosis

Acid-Base Table

Low	Low normal	Normal	High normal	High
				pH 7.48 (alkali)
		pCO2 40 mmHg, 5.3 kPa	Expected pCO2 42 mmHg, 5.6 kPa	
			HCO3 27 mmol	

The table depicts a small uncompensated acute metabolic alkalosis.

Compensation

Expected respiratory compensation is:

$$pCO_2 = 0.6 * (HCO_3^- - 24) + 40 = 42 \text{ mmHg}$$

which is close to the patient's pCO2 of 40 mmHg. These figures are not significantly abnormal, but it would be expected that pCO2 will rise, as compensation for the HCO3-, unless the HCO3- falls into the normal range. As it stands, this is an **uncompensated metabolic alkalosis**.

√ √ √ √ √ √ √

8: Metabolic Acidosis

Metabolic acidosis is an increased acid level, due to acid ingestion, increased acid production, decreased acid excretion, GI (gastrointestinal) or renal losses. The acidosis is indicated by a pH lower than 7.4, and HCO3- lower than 22 mmol/litre, that is caused either by a failure of the kidneys to remove H+ ions, a build-up of acidity due to sepsis, ketones (DKA), lactate, uraemia, heart failure, drugs, aspirin overdose, cardiac arrest, or ingestion of toxins. The acid-base imbalance can also be caused by loss of bicarbonate (HCO3-) due to e.g. pancreatic fistula, or diarrhoea, and calculation of the Anion Gap (Appendix 8) can point to whether or not this loss is the cause of the acidosis. Treatment might include sodium bicarbonate.

Identifying the metabolic imbalance is as straight forward as with respiratory cases, except that it is the bicarbonate (HCO3-) level that indicates the acid/alkali state, and it is a decrease in HCO3- that suggests acidity, as opposed to increased carbon dioxide of a respiratory acidosis.

Another difference from respiratory acid-base recognition is that of the calculation from expected compensation that occurs with metabolic cases. Specifically, the expected respiratory CO2 compensation in a metabolic acidosis is described by Winter's Formula:

$$pCO_2 = (1.5 * HCO_3^-) + 8 \text{ mmHg } (+/- 2)$$

As ever, examples, repetition, and experience produce comprehension.

Of the four different acid-base imbalances, metabolic acidosis is probably the most interesting, because it has associated techniques that make it possible to determine finely grained information about the nature of the disturbance, and whether or not there are additional disturbances that are otherwise not so easy to learn by other means. Specifically, it is use of the Anion Gap (Appendix 8) calculation that is the basis for determining the two main classes of metabolic acidosis, which are of the Normal (NAGMA) and High Anion Gap (HAGMA) types. Additionally, there are the Delta Ratio and Delta Gap calculations, which give extra evidence of what mixed disturbances exist, and the causes of such.

Examples

The following first three examples are straight forward, and should be quite easy to understand for the reader who has read thus far, and are probably at a sufficient level of difficulty necessary for most nursing staff. After that, the examples become more complex. Understanding these more complex scenarios is, of course, desirable, but not essential for most nurses, and they are certainly closer to the description of "And A Little More" than "The Basics", so don't worry if they are too confusing or, indeed, at a level of complexity that is unnecessary for your role, in which case, skip over those examples, and stick with the basics!

√ √ √ √ √ √ √

Example 13

Entity	Value	Normal Range
pO2	10.5 kPa (79 mmHg)	10–13.3 kPa (75-100 mmHg)
SO2	95%	95-100%
pH	7.25 ↓	7.35–7.45
pCO2	5.2 kPa (39 mmHg)	4.7–6 kPa (35-45 mmHg)
HCO3-	18 mmol/L ↓	22-26 mmol/L

Oxygenation

Oxygen partial pressure (pO2) and saturation (HCO3-) are in the normal range.

Acid-Base

pH of 7.25 is an acidaemia.

Carbon Dioxide (pCO2)

CO2 is very normal, which is the first clue that this is NOT a primary respiratory disturbance.

Bicarbonate (HCO3-)

HCO3- of 18 mmol is acidic, so this is a metabolic acidosis.

8: Metabolic Acidosis

Acid-Base Table

Low	Low normal	Normal	High normal	High
pH 7.25 (acid)				
	pCO_2 39 mmHg, (*Expected* 35 mmHg)			
HCO_3^- 18 mmol (acid)				

Low pH and HCO_3^- confirm metabolic acidosis.

Compensation

Expected CO_2 compensation:

$$pCO_2 = (1.5 * HCO_3) + 8,$$
$$pCO_2 = (1.5 * \mathbf{18}) + 8 = 35 \text{ mmHg } (+/- 2)$$

With a blood gas pCO_2 of 39 mmHg, either is no respiratory compensation occurring, making this a mixed **metabolic and respiratory acidosis** (Appendix 3, rule 1).

√ √ √ √ √ √ √

Example 14

Entity	Value	Normal Range
pO_2	11.5 kPa (86 mmHg)	10–13.3 kPa (75-100 mmHg)
SO_2	96%	95-100%
pH	7.33 ↓	7.35–7.45
pCO_2	4.1 kPa ↓ (31 mmHg)	4.7–6 kPa (35-45 mmHg)
HCO_3^-	18 mmol/L ↓	22-26 mmol/L

Oxygenation
pO_2 and SO_2 are normal.

Acid-Base
pH of 7.33 is very slightly acidic (acidaemia).

Carbon Dioxide (pCO_2)
CO_2 of 31 mmHg (4.1 kPa) is low, and could be either due to a little hyperventilation, or compensation for metabolic acidosis.

Bicarbonate (HCO_3)
HCO_3^- of 18 mmol and the low pH suggest metabolic acidosis. CO_2 of 31 mmHg (4.1 kPa) is low, and could be either due to a little hyperventilation, or compensation for metabolic acidosis.

8: Metabolic Acidosis

Acid-Base Table

	Low	Low normal	Normal	High normal	High
pH 7.33 (acid)					
pCO2 31 mmHg, 4.1 kPa (alkali)		Expected pCO2 35 mmHg, 4.7 kPa			
HCO3- 18 mmol (acid)					

The above pattern is clearly of a metabolic acidosis, with partial respiratory compensation.

Compensation

Expected CO2 compensation:

$$pCO2 = (1.5 * HCO3^-) + 8 = 35 \text{ mmHg } (+/- 2),$$

$$pCO2 = (1.5 * 18) + 8 = 35 \text{ mmHg } (+/- 2)$$

The pCO2 of 31 mmHg is lower than what the expected value suggests but, with a tolerance between 33-37 mmHg, this might be defined as a **partially compensated metabolic acidosis** (Appendx 3, rule 2). Alternatively, there may also be a simultaneous small **respiratory alkalosis** present. Note: with this single snapshot that the blood gas gives, it is not possible to be definitive about which is the true acid-base status, but other information, including patterns revealed from previous blood gases, may make the picture clearer.

Example 15

Entity	Value	Normal Range
pO_2	12.7 kPa (96 mmHg)	10–13.3 kPa (75-100 mmHg)
SO_2	97%	95-100%
pH	7.35	7.35–7.45
pCO_2	4.4 kPa ↓ (33 mmHg)	4.7–6 kPa (35-45 mmHg)
HCO_3^-	16 mmol/L ↓	22-26 mmol/L

Oxygenation
Both pO_2 and SO_2 are normal.

Acid-Base
pH 7.35 is just inside the low side of the normal range.

Carbon Dioxide (pCO_2)
CO_2 of 33 mmHg (4.4 kPa) suggests compensation for a metabolic acidosis, and will be proved/disproved by the compensation calculation.

Bicarbonate (HCO_3^-)
HCO_3^- of 16 mmol is an acidotic value, suggesting metabolic acidosis.

Acid-Base Table

Low	Low normal	Normal	High normal	High
	pH 7.35			
pCO2 33 mmHg, 4.4 kPa (alkali) *Expected 32 mmHg*				
HCO3- 16 mmol (acid)				

The table gives a good graphical reflection of a fully compensated metabolic acidosis (Appendix 3, rule 2).

Compensation

Expected CO_2 compensation:

$$pCO_2 = (1.5 * \mathbf{16}) + 8 = 32 \text{ mmHg } (+/- 2)$$

32 mmHg closely "matches" the patient's pCO2 of 33 mmHg, and gives further evidence of a **compensated metabolic acidosis**.

√ √ √ √ √ √ √

Example 16

This example is a step up in complexity, and is meant to introduce some of the techniques that anaesthetists use to reveal details about a blood gas assay.

Entity	Value	Normal Range
pO_2	11.3 kPa (85 mmHg)	10–13.3 kPa (75-100 mmHg)
SO_2	96%	95-100%
pH	7.4	7.35–7.45
pCO_2	5.4 kPa (41 mmHg)	4.7–6 kPa (35-45 mmHg)
HCO_3^-	22 mmol/L	22-26 mmol/L
Na^+	143 mmol/L	133-146 mmol/L
Cl^-	92 mmol/L ↓	95-108 mmol/L
K^+	3.3 mmol/L ↓	3.5-5.3 mmol/L

Oxygenation

There values for pO_2 and oxygen saturation are normal for a patient breathing room air.

Acid-Base

pH of 7.4 is a biological neutral value – neither acidic or alkalotic, so might be described as "perfect".

8: Metabolic Acidosis

Carbon Dioxide (pCO2)
CO2 of 41 mmHg (5.4 kPa) is very normal.

Bicarbonate (HCO3-)
HCO3- of 22 mmol/L is on the low (acidic) side of normal.

Acid-Base Table

Low	Low normal	Normal	High normal	High
		pH 7.4		
			pCO2 41 mmHg, 5.4 kPa	
	HCO3- 22 mmol			

Apparently, there are no acid-base disturbances.

Compensation
The acid-base values are too confusing to decide what, if any, the primary disturbance is, so compensation calculations are inappropriate, because pH is the "neutral" value of 7.4. Anion Gap calculations will have to be used to determine what disturbance(s) may be occurring.

Anion Gap (AG)
Anion Gap distinguishes between the two types of metabolic acidosis: Normal Anion Gap (NAGMA, 8-16) and High Anion Gap (HAGMA, > 16).

Calculating 143 (N+) − 92 (Cl-) -22 (HCO3-) = **29**, which is a HAGMA (high anion gap metabolic acidosis).

Delta Ratio (DR)

DR is the Anion Gap difference from normal, divided by HCO_3^- difference from normal: (29-12) / (24-22) = 17/2 = 8.5, which meets the definition (see Glossary) for mixed **high anion gap metabolic acidosis and metabolic alkalosis.**

Note: the slightly low potassium (K+) level supports the conclusion that a metabolic alkalosis exists.

Delta Gap

To support the Delta Ratio conclusion, the Delta Gap (Glossary) value of 15 (17-2) also suggests **high anion gap metabolic acidosis and metabolic alkalosis.**

Note that this artificial example is intended to illustrate how an apparently normal looking acid-base balance, with perfect pH, can actually hide disturbances that are only revealed with the above basic Anion Gap calculations.

√ √ √ √ √ √ √

Example 17

Entity	Value	Normal Range
pO2	12.1 kPa (91 mmHg)	30 kPa (**30% FiO2**) (226 mmHg)
SO2	98%	95-100%
pH	7.25 ↓	7.35–7.45
pCO2	4.2 kPa ↓ (32 mmHg)	4.7–6 kPa (35-45 mmHg)
HCO3-	12 mmol/L ↓	22-26 mmol/L
Na+	145 mmol/L	133-146 mmol/L
K+	2 mmol/L ↓	3.5-5.3 mmol/L
Cl-	96 mmol/L	95-108 mmol/L
Glucose	15 mmol/L ↑	4-7 mmol/L

The patient is a Type 1 diabetic.

Oxygenation

The pO2 of 91 mmHg (12.1 kPa) and 98% SO2 seem fine, but the patient is intubated, and pO2 should be 10 kPa less than the FiO2: 30-10 = 20 kPa, so a pO2 of 12.1 kPa suggests a ventilation or perfusion problem.

P/F Ratio

Divide pO2 (mmHg) by FiO2: 91/0.3 = **303**. Despite the good oxygenation status, the low P/F Ratio of 303 shows that the patient might have lung damage, inflammation, or Acute Respiratory Distress

Syndrome. If the patient was breathing room air, pO2 would be 0.21 * 303 = 64 mmHg, which is close to the value (60 mmHg) that describes respiratory failure. After extubation, the patient might need continued ventilation support.

Acid-Base
pH of 7.25 is acidic.

Carbon Dioxide (pCO2)
CO2 of 32 mmHg (4.2 kPa) is slightly on the alkalotic side of the normal range.

Bicarbonate (HCO3-)
HCO3- of 12 mmol/L is acidotic, and corresponds with the pH for a primary metabolic acidosis.

Glucose
The patient is a Type 1 diabetic, and a glucose level of 15 mmol/litre suggests diabetic ketoacidosis, so an Anion Gap calculation will probably reveal a high anion gap metabolic acidosis (HAGMA).

Acid-Base Table

Low	Low normal	Normal	High normal	High
pH 7.25 (acid)				
pCO2 32 mmHg, 4.2 kPa (*Expected* 26 mmHg)				
HCO3- 12 mmol (acid)				

This pattern depicts a part compensated metabolic acidosis.

Compensation

Expected CO2 compensation:

$$pCO_2 = (1.5 * HCO_3^-) + 8 = mmHg (+/- 2)$$
$$pCO_2 = (1.5 * \mathbf{12}) + 8 = 26 \text{ mmHg}$$

The patient's pCO2 of 32 mmHg is higher than the expected value of 26 mmHg, which means there may be a respiratory acidosis present.

Anion Gap (AG, Appendix 8)

Sodium – chloride – bicarbonate --> Na+ - Cl- - HCO3- -->

145 – 96 – 12 = **37**, which is 25 above normal, so this is a HAGMA (high anion gap metabolic acidosis).

Delta (Δ) Ratio

AG (Anion Gap) is 25 above normal, and HCO3- is 12 below normal. Delta Ratio is 25/12 = **2.1**, which suggests HAGMA plus metabolic alkalosis, where the HAGMA is probably due to the diabetic ketoacidosis – so the patient might need intravenous fluids and insulin. Note the low potassium level is an extra sign of a metabolic alkalosis.

Conclusion: The patient needs management for diabetes mellitus, has a ventilation and/or perfusion problem, and a triple acid-base disturbance of metabolic acidosis (diabetic ketoacidosis), plus metabolic alkalosis and a respiratory acidosis.

√ √ √ √ √ √ √

8: Metabolic Acidosis

Example 18

Entity	Value	Normal Range
pO2	11 kPa (83 mmHg)	10–13.3 kPa (75-100 mmHg)
SO2	95%	95-100%
pH	7.27 ↓	7.35–7.45
pCO2	5.4 kPa (41 mmHg)	4.7–6 kPa (35-45 mmHg)
HCO3-	14 mmol/L ↓	22-26 mmol/L
Na+	140 mmol/L	133-146 mmol/L
K+	4 mmol/L	3.5-5.3 mmol/L
Cl-	105 mmol/L	95-108 mmol/L

Oxygenation

SO2 (95%) and pO2 (11 kPa, 83 mmHg) are normal.

Acid-Base

pH of 7.27 is acidic.

Carbon Dioxide (pCO2)

CO2 of 41 mmHg (5.4 kPa) is very normal, so the acidosis must be metabolic (HCO3-).

Bicarbonate (HCO3-)

HCO3- of 14 mmol/litre confirms a metabolic acidosis.

Acid-Base Table

Low	Low normal	Normal	High normal	High
pH 7.27 (acid)				
Expected pCO2 29 mmHg, 3.9 kPa			pCO2 41 mmHg, 5.4 kPa	
HCO3- 14 mmol (acid)				

The table suggests an uncompensated metabolic acidosis.

Compensation

Expected CO_2 compensation:

$$pCO_2 = (1.5 * HCO_3^-) + 8 = \text{mmHg} (+/- 2)$$
$$pCO_2 = (1.5 * 14) + 8 = \mathbf{29} \text{ mmHg}$$

The patient's pCO_2 of 41 mmHg, is higher than the expected 29 mmHg, which probably means there is a respiratory acidosis in progress - check the Delta Ratio.

Anion Gap (AG, Appendix 8)

AG = 140 (N+) − 105 (Cl-) − 14 (HCO3-) = **21**, which is 9 above normal (12), so this is probably a HAGMA (high anion gap metabolic acidosis).

Delta Ratio (see Glossary)

Use the delta ratio to find more in depth information about the metabolic acidosis: AG is 9 above normal, and HCO3- is 10 below normal. Delta Ratio is 9/10 = **0.9**, which suggests mixed normal and high Anion Gap metabolic acidosis (caused by lactic acidosis, diabetic acidosis, OR inability to eliminate acids due to kidney failure).

Conclusion

In the absence of further information, this appears to be a **mixed normal (NAGMA) and high (HAGMA) Anion Gap metabolic acidosis, plus a possible respiratory acidosis.**

√ √ √ √ √ √ √

Example 19

Entity	Value	Normal Range
pO2	8.6 kPa ↓ (66 mmHg)	10–13.3 kPa (75-100 mmHg)
SO2	91% ↓	95-100%
pH	7.3 ↓	7.35–7.45
pCO2	4.7 kPa (35 mmHg)	4.7–6 kPa (35-45 mmHg)
HCO3-	10 mmol/L ↓	22-26 mmol/L
Na+	138 mmol/L	133-146 mmol/L
K+	5.5 mmol/L ↑	3.5-5.3 mmol/L
Cl-	107 mmol/L	95-108 mmol/L

Note: This is more complicated than it first appears.

Oxygenation

Oxygen partial pressure of 66 mmHg (8.6 kPa) and 91% saturation are hypoxic values. The patient needs supplementary oxygen.

Acid-Base

pH of 7.3 is low, and is acidaemic.

Carbon Dioxide (pCO2)

CO2 of 35 mmHg (4.7 kPa) is a little low, so is possibly compensating for the acidaemia – more time maybe?

Bicarbonate (HCO3-)

HCO3- of 10 mmol/L is acidic, so this is a metabolic acidotic condition.

Acid-Base Table

Low	Low normal	Normal	High normal	High
pH 7.3 (acid)				
Expected pCO2 23 mmHg	pCO2 35 mmHg, 4.7 kPa			
HCO3- 10 mmol (acid)				

The pattern reflects the earlier assumption that this is a metabolic acidosis, with some compensation.

Compensation

Expected CO_2 compensation:

$$pCO_2 = (1.5 * HCO_3^-) + 8 = mmHg (+/- 2)$$
$$pCO_2 = (1.5 * \mathbf{10}) + 8 = 23\ mmHg$$

The expected pCO2 of 23 mmHg (4 kPa) is lower than the patient value of 35 mmHg (4.7 kPa), so there appears to be both metabolic and respiratory acidosis occurring.

Hyperkalaemia

The slightly high potassium (K) of 5.5 mmol/litre must be investigated for the cause, which might be endocrine issues, kidney failure, or drugs. (Insulin and dextrose may be needed?)

Anion Gap & Delta Ratio

AG = 134 − 103 − 10 = **21**, which is 9 higher than normal, so this might be a HAGMA (high anion gap metabolic acidosis). Delta Ratio is 9 divided by HCO3- difference from normal: 9/14 = **0.6**, which means **combined respiratory, HAGMA, and NAGMA metabolic acidosis.**

This example demonstrates that the interpretation of the acid-base values (pH, pCO2, HCO3-), such as described from the above Acid-Base Table, do not always reflect the underlying problems as well as the Anion Gap values do.

√ √ √ √ √ √ √

9: Case Study

Entity	Value	Normal Range
pO2	7.4 kPa ↓ (on CPAP) (56 mmHg)	10–13.3 kPa (75-100 mmHg)
SO2	51% ↓	95-100%
pH	6.72 ↓	7.35–7.45
pCO2	13.4 kPa ↑ (101 mmHg)	4.7–6 kPa (35-45 mmHg)
HCO3-	13 mmol/L ↓	22-26 mmol/L
Glucose	13.6 mmol/L ↑	3.6-5.3 mmol/L
Lactate	15 mmol/L ↑	0.5-2.2 mmol/L
Potassium	5.9 mmol/L (K+) ↑	3.5-5.3 mmol/L

Oxygenation

Both pO2 and O2 saturation are low, even though the patient is supported by CPAP. Intubation is probably needed, so an anaesthetist should be called for – with urgency! Then, other checks should be made of Hb, haematocrit, carbon monoxide poisoning, and anything that helps build a picture of the problems this patient is experiencing: The high lactate suggests anaerobic metabolism - so probable lactic acidosis, and sepsis - and the high glucose is indicative of diabetic ketoacidosis. (Note: the high potassium level can result in cardiac arrest)

Acid-Base
pH of 6.72 may not be survivable.

Carbon Dioxide (pCO2)
The very high CO2 is indicative of a serious ventilation and/or perfusion problem, with a dangerous degree of CO2 retention, and is clear evidence of respiratory acidosis. Together with the low pO2 level, this reveals a Respiratory Failure, Type II (hypercapnic).

Bicarbonate (HCO3-)
13 mmol/litre corresponds with a metabolic acidosis.

Compensation
Working out the compensation is pointless; this patient is near death!

Acid-Base Table

Low	Low normal	Normal	High normal	High
pH 6.72 (acid)				
				pCO2 101 mmHg, 13.4 kPa (acid)

Low	Low normal	Normal	High normal	High
HCO3⁻ 13 mmol (acid)				

This is a pattern of mixed respiratory and metabolic acidosis.

Glucose

The high glucose of 13.6 mmol/litre probably means that tissue damage is occurring, and the damage to blood vessels is increasing the risk of myocardial infarction and nervous system problems.

Lactate

Lactate of 15 mmol/litre is serious (dehydration, anaemia, sepsis?).

Background

This is the case of a 6 day old baby, who was brought to the emergency unit of Chelsea & Westminster Hospital in 2015, and admitted to the High Dependency Unit just before 20:00. Blood gases were taken at: 20:38 (pH=**7.28**), 01:32 (pH=**7.06**), 04:10 (pH=**6.72**), and 05:00 (pH=**6.69**). The baby breathed room air, until 02:00, then Optiflow until 03:00, then CPAP at 03:00. The assay is from the 04:10 blood gas.

Even though ALL indications pointed to the necessity of intubation, and treating the baby as an emergency case, which is what it was, the Consultant Paediatrician took no interest - he was preoccupied with his girlfriend, who was the nurse assigned to care for the baby. Shortly after starting her night shift, the nurse told the parents that she was leaving the unit, and would monitor the child remotely. There was no remote monitoring facility. The nurse went to spend the night in her

9: Case Study

boyfriend's (Paediatrician) office, which they locked. The baby's parents were at their baby's cotside, for the whole of the night.

From the time of admission, the duty Registrar, and the Consultant, recorded the baby as in respiratory distress, and ventilatory failure, with respiratory rate of 48, but no decision was made to use supplementary oxygen, until 03:00, when Optiflow was applied.

The lactate and glucose problems were not addressed, and no attempt was made to put the baby on the sepsis protocol or, indeed, to follow the hospital's own protocols for dealing with such a case.

The other nurses on duty were concerned about the baby, but didn't have the blood gas interpretation skills to recognise how serious the situation was, and were too frightened of the Consultant to use their initiative to call for a senior Anaesthetist to review the baby. Had they done so, and described the blood gas results over the phone, it is almost certain that an Anaesthetist would have attended, the case would have been escalated to Intensive Care, and the baby would have survived. Unfortunately, if the nurses had taken it upon themselves to side-step the Consultant, the nurses would have suffered retribution and resultant career termination, because that is the culture of the doctor:nurse relationship - nurses should never disagree with a doctor. Incidentally, two other junior doctors also reviewed the baby's condition, but they too had to bow to the seniority of the Consultant.

The baby died, of cardiac arrest, at 05:45.

If any one of the nurses had the basic blood gas interpretation skills, perhaps gained from a book such as this, and used that knowledge to demand the attendence of an Anaesthetist, Intensivist, or even the Crash Team, she/he could have, at least, used that knowledge to justify their actions on the basis of complying with the Precautionary

Principle, which is a tenet of the British safety culture, as described by the Health and Safety at Work Act duty to reduce risk.

The question that you, as a nurse or allied health professional, must ask, is "Would I have sacrificed my career in the attempt to save the life of this baby, or would I have followed the chain of command and let others dictate events?"

√ √ √ √ √ √ √

10: Self Test

Q 1. What disturbance is signified by these values:

pH:	7.23
pCO2:	7.7 kPa (58 mmHg)
HCO3-:	30 mmol/litre

Q 2. In what practical way does a "normal" Anion Gap metabolic acidosis (NAGMA) differ from a "high" Anion Gap metabolic acidosis (HAGMA)?

Q 3. If haemoglobin (Hb) is low, SO2 (oxygen saturation) will also be low. True or false?

Q 4. How does nasogastric suctioning affect acid-base balance?

Q 5. If a respiratory acidosis is partially compensated, pH will be lower than 7.35. True or false?

Q 6. What disturbance is signified by these values:

| pH: | 7.24 |

pCO2:	8.8 kPa (66 mmHg)
HCO3-:	40 mmol/litre

Q 7. The patient has hypoxia, and mixed respiratory and metabolic acidosis. Which blood gas set indicates this?

SET	pO2	pH	pCO2	HCO3-
1	9.3 kPa (70 mmHg)	7.15	6.5 kPa (49 mmHg)	28 mmol
2	9.3 kPa (70 mmHg)	7.15	6.5 kPa (49 mmHg)	10 mmol
3	7.5 kPa (56 mmHg)	7.15	4 kPa (30 mmHg)	28 mmol
4	7.5 kPa (56 mmHg)	7.15	4 kPa (30 mmHg)	10 mmol

Q 8. A low albumin count can make a normal anion gap metabolic acidosis appear like a high anion gap metabolic acidosis. True or false?

Q 9. What disturbance is signified by these values:

pH:	7.39
pCO2:	4.8 kPa (36 mmHg)
HCO3-:	18 mmol/litre

Q 10. What are typical symptoms/signs for respiratory acidosis?

Q 11. It is not possible for a patient to simultaneously have respiratory acidosis and respiratory alkalosis. True or false?

10: Self Test

Q 12. What is the normal link between pO2 and FiO2?

Q 13. A blood gas assay shows Type I respiratory failure and partially compensated respiratory alkalosis. Which set of blood gas values reflect this condition?

SET	pO2	pH	pCO2	HCO3-
1	7.5 kPa (56 mmHg)	7.55	4 kPa (30 mmHg)	20 mmol
2	7.5 kPa (56 mmHg)	7.55	8 kPa (60 mmHg)	20 mmol
3	7.5 kPa (56 mmHg)	7.25	4 kPa (30 mmHg)	28 mmol
4	7.5 kPa (56 mmHg)	7.25	8 kPa (60 mmHg)	28 mmol

Q 14. How does a change in Minute Volume alter acid status?

Q 15. Vomiting can cause loss of bicarbonate, with resultant acidosis. True or false?

Q 16. What disturbance is signified by these values:

pH:	7.22
pCO2:	3.3 kPa (25 mmHg)
HCO3-:	12 mmol/litre
Na+:	140 mmol/litre
K+:	4.5 mmol/litre
Cl-:	97

10: Self Test

Q 17. The patient is experiencing mixed metabolic and respiratory alkalosis. Which blood gas set indicates this?

SET	pO2	pH	pCO2	HCO3-
1	7.3 kPa (55 mmHg)	7.15	6.5 kPa (49 mmHg)	19 mmol
2	7.3 kPa (55 mmHg)	7.15	6.5 kPa (49 mmHg)	29 mmol
3	12 kPa (90 mmHg)	7.6	3.7 kPa (28 mmHg)	19 mmol
4	12 kPa (90 mmHg)	7.6	3.7 kPa (28 mmHg)	29 mmol

Q 18. If a respiratory acidosis is partially compensated, pH will be lower than 7.35. True or false?

Q 19. What does Anion Gap mean?

Q 20. What is the most common cause of metabolic acidosis?

Q 21. Carbon monoxide (CO) poisoning causes low paO2 (arterial oxygen partial pressure). True or false?

Q 22. To convert kPa to mmHg, multiply the kPa by 7.4. True or false?

Q 23. The patient has Type 2 respiratory failure and partially compensated respiratory acidosis, which set of blood gas values reflect this condition?

10: Self Test

SET	pO2	pH	pCO2	HCO3-
1	7 kPa (53 mmHg)	7.18	5.7 kPa (43 mmHg)	30 mmol
2	10 kPa (75 mmHg)	7.5	5.7 kPa (43 mmHg)	18 mmol
3	7 kPa (53 mmHg)	7.18	8.7 kPa (65 mmHg)	30 mmol
4	10 kPa (75 mmHg)	7.5	8.7 kPa (65 mmHg)	18 mmol

Q 24. What disturbance is signified by these values:

pH:	7.57
pCO2:	3.6 kPa (27 mmHg)
HCO3-:	21 mmol/litre

Q 25. What acid-base disturbance is indicated by this panel?

	Low	Low normal	Normal	High normal	High
	pCO2 29 mmHg, 3.8 kPa (alkali)		HCO3- 24 mmol		pH 7.5 (alkali)

√ √ √ √ √ √ √

11: Self Test Answers

A 1. Partially compensated respiratory acidosis.

A 2. A normal AG metabolic acidosis is due to loss of bicarbonate – compensated by high chloride levels – caused by loss from the GI tract (eg, diarrhoea), renal tubular acidosis, or displacement of bicarbonate by intravenous sodium chloride.

A 3. False; SO_2 level is determined by the fraction of Hb that are fully bound with oxygen – not the total oxygen carried by the Hb.

A 4. Suctioning removes enough H+ ions to produce a metabolic alkalaemia. Severe vomiting and diuretics have a similar effect.

A 5. True. When fully compensated, pH will be at least 7.35, but below 7.4.

A 6. Mixed respiratory acidosis and metabolic alkalosis.

A 7. Set 2: Hypoxia, and mixed respiratory and metabolic acidosis.

11: Self Test Answers

A 8. False. Low albumin can make a HAGMA appear as a NAGMA.

A 9. Compensated metabolic acidosis.

A 10. Breathing difficulty, hypoventilation, confusion, tachycardia, headache, low pH, high paCO2.

A 11. True. Respiratory acidosis and respiratory alkalosis cannot occur together.

A 12. pO2 (kPa) should be ~ FiO2 % - 10.

A 13. Set 1: Type I respiratory failure and partially compensated respiratory alkalosis.

A 14. An increase in Minute Volume, either by increasing respiratory rate or Tidal Volume, increases expiration of CO2, and so reduces acidity (H+ ion concentration), and increases pH. A decrease in Minute Volume causes CO2 retention, and increases acidity – lowering pH.

A 15. False. Vomiting causes loss of H+ ions, with resultant alkalosis.

A 16. Partially compensated metabolic acidosis: Anion Gap is 31, so this is a high anion gap metabolic acidosis (HAGMA). Note: Delta Gap suggests there may also be a metabolic alkalosis.

A 17. Set 4: Mixed metabolic and respiratory alkalosis.

A 18. True. When fully compensated, pH will be at least 7.35, but below 7.4.

11: Self Test Answers

A 19. The difference between unmeasured cations and unmeasured anions, measured indirectly by subtracting measured anions from measured cations. A smaller anion gap suggests loss of bicarbonate, whereas a higher anion gap number signifies excess H+ ions.

A 20. High lactate level, producing lactic acidosis. Usually, high lactate is due to oxygenation problems, and the high lactate is a reliable indicator of sepsis. The liver is the main organ for clearing lactate, so liver problems can also cause high levels of lactate.

A 21. False. CO does not affect paO2, but does prevent oxygen from binding with Hb, because CO binds more easily with Hb than does oxygen, so causing reduced oxygen available for oxygenation of the tissues.

A 22. False; multiply kPa by 7.5 to get mmHg.

A 23. Set 3: Type 2 respiratory failure and partially compensated respiratory acidosis.

A 24. Partially compensated respiratory alkalosis.

A 25. Uncompensated respiratory alkalosis, typically due to hyperventilation. This is, presumably, an acute condition, because the kidneys have not had time to start compensation with HCO3-.

√ √ √ √ √ √ √

Appendix 1: Glossary

Appendix 1: Glossary

Definitions from *Glossary of Anaesthetics* (Amazon Publishing)

Acidaemia

Acidity means an aqueous solution has a pH below 7 but, in healthcare, acidity refers to a pH lower than 7.4, which is the optimum value for the body, even though pH above 7 is, technically, alkaline. Acidaemia means an acid (excess H+ ions) state of the blood, either because the kidneys (metabolic acidosis) are not eliminating H+, or the lungs (respiratory acidosis) are not eliminating enough CO_2. Some factors that cause acidity include: high pCO_2, high Cl-, and albumin. Acidifying factors include high values for CO_2, Cl, and albumin. Acidaemia causes vasoconstriction.

Acidity

The level of H+ ion concentration ([H+]), as measured by the pH scale. Acid build-up can be caused by hypoventilation, sepsis, ketones, toxins,

Appendix 1: Glossary

and ingestion of acids. Acidity can be reduced by severe vomiting, or acid removal from the stomach by NG suctioning.

Acidosis

True acidosis means pH is below 7, but blood acidotic conditions are values below 7.4, and are properly referred to as *physiological acidosis*. In blood gas analysis, acidosis refers to the process that creates the acidaemia. Note: a patient may have an "acidosis" process in progress, but compensation may push pH into the normal range, thereby disguising the acidosis. Acidosis reduces alveolar uptake of oxygen.

Acute Ventilatory Failure

Type II respiratory failure: inability to clear CO_2, with resultant low pH, usually due to hypoventilation, which causes a low arterial oxygen pressure (pO_2). Giving oxygen does not fix the problem - intubate instead, and address the hypoventilation problem.

Acute Alveolar Hyperventilation

Hyperventilation caused by hypoxaemia, measured by arterial oxygen pressure (pO_2), and signified by: high (alkalotic) pH, low CO_2, normal bicarbonate (HCO_3^-). Give oxygen.

Alkaline

See Base.

Albumin

The major unmeasured anion : A weak acidic protein, made by the liver, that serves to keep fluid in the bloodstream, and transports enzymes, vitamins, hormones, around the body. A low level of albumin means more space for bicarbonate in the blood, and so low albumin is associated with alkalosis. Hypoalbuminaemia can also be a sign of malnutrition, liver disease, or kidney disease. High albumin means less bicarbonate, so has an acidic effect. See *Anion Gap*.

Alkalosis/Alkalaemia

Alkalaemia (pH > 7.45) means an excessive base of the blood, indicated by a high level of buffers (eg, bicarbonate), or reduced acidity. **Alkalosis** refers to the process that creates the alkalaemia. Factors that increase alkalaemia are low values for CO_2 and Cl.

Anaemia

The inability of blood to transport a normal amount of oxygen, either because of a deficient amount of Hb, or some of the Hb is defective (or bound wth carbon monoxide). Note that a patient can have insufficient Hb to allow proper tissue oxygenation, but a normal SO_2 level, because SO_2 concerns the amount of oxygen molecules that are bound to Hb, as a fraction of oxygen molecule that could be bound to Hb.

A simile would be a group of 10 buses that collectively carry 300 passengers, out of a total capacity of 400 passengers (40 per bus), so the group of buses is 75% loaded (saturated). If there were another group of only 2 buses, with all 80 seats taken, they would be 100% loaded (saturated), which is a higher % than the group of 10 buses, but they are carrying a smaller number of passengers. It is the same with Hb - if there are not enough Hb molecules available to allow normal oxygenation (anaemic), but every Hb molecule is fully loaded with its maximum of 4 oxygen molecules, SO_2 would be 100%, even though the amount of O_2 is too low for proper oxygenation.

Appendix 1: Glossary

Anion

A negatively charged ion (atom, molecule, compound) - more electrons than protons. Chloride and bicarbonate constitute 85% of the body's anions, and their values help determine the Anion Gap.

Anion Gap (AG)

The difference between unmeasured anions and unmeasured cations, derived from the calculation of sodium − chloride − bicarbonate, with a normal value (assuming normal albumin) of 12 mmol/litre (142−105−25) +/- 4. During metabolic acidosis, an Anion Gap calculation helps find the cause, which might be loss of bicarbonate, such as due to diarrhoea or renal tubular acidosis, in which case there will be a *hyperchloraemic acidosis*. An AG above 30 mmol is a high AG metabolic acidosis (HAGMA), and is commonly caused by TRKL (Toxin ingestion, Renal failure, Ketoacidosis, or Lactic acidosis). If AG is 20 mmol/litre, there is a 30% chance of a high anion gap metabolic acidosis (HAGMA) being present, climbing to almost 100% when AG reaches 30. See *NAGMA, HAGMA, Appendix 8.*

Atom

An atom is the smallest particle that can normally exist on its own. There are 92 different types of atom that occur naturally, and these are known as elements. In the body, atom types, or elements, include sodium (Na), nitrogen (symbol N), oxygen (O), carbon (C), hydrogen (H), potassium (K), chlorine (Cl), and many others.

Every atom has a nucleus, containing at least 1 proton, which is positively charged, at least 1 neutron (except hydrogen), which has no charge, and 1 or more electrons, which are negatively charged.

In any atom, the number of protons determines what element it is. For

Appendix 1: Glossary

example, if an atom has only 1 proton, it is a hydrogen atom; if an atom contains 8 protons, it is an oxygen atom. The number of protons gives each element its identifying number, known as "Atomic Number", and its place on the Periodic Table (later).

Atomic Mass

More formally, *Relative Atomic Mass*, old term *Atomic Weight*: The number that indicates the mass of 1 mole of the particular element, in grams, and is derived from the total protons added to the mean number of neutrons. Carbon, for example, symbol "C", has 6 protons and an average 6.01 neutrons, so 1 mole of carbon atoms has weighs (atomic mass) 6 + 6.01 = 12.01 g.

Base

A substance that can neutralise an acid, forming a salt, when in solution, by accepting H+ (positive hydrogen) ions (protons). In the blood, the bicarbonate (cation) base is the body's most important buffer that accepts (mops up) H+ ions. If the base dissolves in water, it is known as an alkali.

Base Excess

A value that is derived from pH and pCO_2 values, where a positive value (usually) means a metabolic alkalotic condition, or a negative value (Base Deficit) that (usually) indicates metabolic acidosis. A positive value describes how much acid (mmol) would have to be added to a litre of the patient's blood (at 37°C, and pCO_2 of 40 mmHg), if pH is to be reduced to a save level of 7.4 {reference to "base" is mostly to bicarbonate (HCO_3-)}. If BE is greater than +2 mmol/L level, the abnormal excess of base in the blood will be caused by metabolic alkalosis, or respiratory compensation. Conversely, if BE is less than -2

Appendix 1: Glossary

mmol/L, the low level will be caused by metabolic acidosis, or a respiratory compensation. Base Excess helps reveal the metabolic component of an acid-base disturbance.

Bicarbonate (HCO3-)

Aka *Hydrogen Carbonate*, calculated from pH and pCO2; a base/alkali ion that is the principle transport mechanism for CO2, and the main buffer for excess hydrogen ions (H+), so maintaining acid-base balance. Excreted or reabsorbed by the kidneys, in response to pH levels. Note: some ABG machines give bicarbonate values in mEq/L, but converting to mmol/L is 1:1, so no conversion has to occur.

Bicarbonate Buffer Equation

$$CO_2 + H_2O \Longleftrightarrow H_2CO_3 \Longleftrightarrow HCO_3^- + H^+$$

The reversible equation that describes how carbonic acid (H2CO3) consumes or releases H+ ions in order to maintain acid-base balance. When CO2 combines with water, carbonic acid is formed, and this can separate into H+ (positive ions) and negative bicarbonate (HCO3-) ions. The process moves the other way when the dissociated carbonic acid and H+ reach the lungs, so that the CO2 can be expired.

Bilirubin

A compound formed from haem, as a waste product when old and defective red blood cells are broken down. A high level gives yellow colour to jaundice, and can occur in trauma or liver problems. Normal range is 1-17 μmol/L.

Buffer

Compounds (weak acid and conjugate base) in the blood that resist fast changes in pH. The main extracellular buffer is bicarbonate (HCO3-); carbonic acid and phosphates are also buffers. A small amount of intracellular buffering also occurs, using proteins (eg, Hb) and phosphate.

Carbaminohaemoglobin (HbCO$_2$)

Hb bound with CO$_2$.

Carbon Dioxide (CO$_2$)

A respiratory acid and metabolic waste product of the oxidisation of sugar in the mitochondria (cellular respiration), which serves to regulate blood pH. Once produced, CO$_2$ molecules are transported in one of three forms: dissolved in plasma, bound to haemoglobin, and carried as part of bicarbonate ion buffering. CO$_2$ is a heavy, colourless, odourless, incombustible, corrosive, and volatile (changes between gas and liquid) compound of carbon and oxygen, which diffuses very quickly from the blood. Of the CO$_2$ produced, ~10% is dissolved in plasma, 10% binds to Hb, and the rest combines with water to form carbonic acid, which then quickly dissociates into hydrogen (H+) and bicarbonate (HCO3-) ions which, in turn, move from blood cells into plasma.

If cardiac output is reduced, end tidal CO$_2$ (EtCO$_2$) may also be reduced. CO$_2$ is a good indicator of respiratory function, and a normal EtCO$_2$ reading is a sign of valid endotracheal tube placement and airway "sealing". When bicarbonate and H+ ions reach the lungs, they recombine to form CO$_2$, and are exhaled. Normal pCO$_2$ is 4.6-6 kPa (35-45 mmHg). Normal pCO$_2$ (alveolar CO$_2$ pressure) is ~0.66 kPa (5 mmHg) lower than pCO$_2$.

Carbonic Acid (H$_2$CO$_3$)

Water combined with carbon dioxide, which then ionises (dissociates) into bicarbonate and a hydrogen ion (H+).

Carboxyhaemoglobin (COHb)

Carbon monoxide (CO) binds with haemoglobin (Hb) much more readily than oxygen, and forms carboxyhaemoglobin (COHb), making it a reversibly defective molecule, and unavailable for carrying oxygen and, if there is a large enough volume of CO, hypoxia may ensue. A normal pO_2 with low SO_2 can be a sign of CO poisoning but, detection of the CO requires a blood gas machine equipped with a CO-oximeter, so may go undetected by less capable machines. For non smokers, < 3% COHb is normal.

Chloride (Cl-)

The most abundant negatively charged electrolyte (anion of chlorine), with levels controlled by the kidneys, serving to maintain fluid balance between the cells and extracellular space, osmotic pressure, hydration, blood pressure, volume, and pH. A **low** level might be associated with low sodium, more space for bicarbonate, and metabolic alkalosis (hypochloraemic alkalosis), caused by: congestive heart failure, metabolic alkalosis, COPD, vomiting, diarrhoea, diuretics, bicarbonate administration, laxatives, steroids, chemotherapy. A **high** level means less space for bicarbonate, and may be associated with metabolic acidosis (hyperchloraemic acidosis), and can be due to high blood sodium (perhaps from administration of too much normal saline, or salt ingestion), kidney disease, reduced albumin, or dehydration, and is associated with respiratory alkalosis. Symptoms include dry mucous membranes, weakness, thirst, and hypertension. Normal serum range is 95 – 108 mmol/litre.

Chloride to Sodium Ratio

Chloride:Sodium (Cl^- : Na^+); a ratio > 80% is acidifying, and a ratio < 72% is alkalinising.

Cl-

See Chloride.

Co-oximeter

A device that measures blood concentration levels of different types of haemoglobin (Hb), namely: oxyhaemoglobin, deoxyhaemoglobin, carboxyhaemoglobin, and methaemoglobin. Unlike simple oximeters, Co-oximeters can differentiate between oxygen and carbon monoxide (CO), and so give more accurate saturation readings.

CO2

Chemical symbol for carbon dioxide.

Compound

Similar to a molecule, but composed of more than one type of atom (element), eg, HCO_3^- (bicarbonate).

Conjugate Base

A base formed after an acid loses a hydrogen ion (H^+). Because it is a base, it can rejoin with the H^+ to assume an acid state again.

ctHb

Total concentration of haemoglobin (Hb) in blood, which includes oxygenated and deoxygenated Hb, plus carboxyhaemoglobin (COHb)

and methaemoglobin (MetHb). Men: 129-166 g/litre. Women: 114-152 g/litre. In anaemic patients, ctHb is lower, but the oxygen saturation value is unaffected.

CtO2

Volume of oxygen dissolved in plasma and bound to haemoglobin, 9-22 ml/100 ml.

Delta (Δ) Gap

Calculation to determine whether a metabolic acidosis is accompanied by another disorder: [Anion Gap (AG) increase from normal] MINUS [bicarbonate (HCO3-) decrease from normal]: (AG-12) − (24-HCO3-), shortens to HCO3- + AG - 36.

Delta Gap	Description
< -6	Rise in Anion Gap is less than fall in bicarbonate, so a NAGMA is also present.
Between -6 and 6	Only a NAGMA is present.
> 6	Increased Anion Gap is greater than the fall in bicarbonate, so a metabolic alkalosis might also be present

See *HAGMA, NAGMA*.

Delta (Δ) Ratio

A calculation to help find the cause of a high Anion Gap metabolic acidosis (HAGMA), and reveal if another acid-base disorder coexists with the HAGMA, by resolving the increase in Anion Gap / decrease in bicarbonate (HCO3-), using the formula: Δ ratio = (AG-12) / (24-

Appendix 1: Glossary

HCO3-):

Ratio	Meaning
< 0.4	A normal-AG metabolic acidosis (hyperchloraemic). {AG is small}
0.4 - 0.9	Mixed NAGMA and HAGMA, with normal kidney function, and acidic anions excreted in urine, as in ketoacidosis or lactic acid (OR kidney failure). {Small difference between HCO3- difference from normal and AG difference from normal}
1 - 2	Pure high-AG metabolic acidosis. {Diff AG > diff HCO3-}
> 2	HAGMA + either metabolic alkalosis or a compensated respiratory acidosis. {Diff AG much > diff HCO3-}

Deoxyhaemoglobin (HHb)

Haemoglobin not bound with oxygen. Former name: Reduced Hb.

Diabetic Ketoacidosis

Metabolic acidotic condition where low levels of insulin, and high glucose, means the DM sufferer cannot utilise enough glucose for energy needs, and causes them to metabolise fat as a substitute, producing high levels of acidic ketones in the bloodstream, as a result. These ketone bodies are used as energy. DK **symptoms** are hypotension, dry mucous membranes, polyuria, breath smell of pear drops or nail varnish, lethargy, need to pee, confusion, vomiting, thirst, tachypnoea, Kussmaul breathing, hyperglycaemia, high ketone level in urine, blood glucose level > 14 mmol/litre, pH < 7.3, HCO3- < 18 mmol/L. **Treatments** include: rehydration and intravenous insulin.

Electrolyte

Ionic minerals found in body fluids and tissues, formed when a

Appendix 1: Glossary

compound (solute) is dissolved in water, and dissociates into its component ions, each of which carries either a positive (cation) or negative (anion) charge, so that the solution becomes electrically conductive. Sodium (Na+) and potassium (K+) are positive electrolytes (cations); chloride (Cl-) and bicarbonate (HCO$_3$-) are negative (anions).

Electron

Outside of an atom's nucleus are the electrons, which have a negative electrical charge. An atom usually has the same number of electrons as protons, in which case the positive (protons) and negative (electrons) charges cancel each other out, leaving the atom with a neutral charge. Unlike the protons and neutrons, however, electrons are not fixed in place, and the atom can gain or lose electrons.

Equivalent (Eq)

A non-SI chemical measurement system, popular in the USA, but not generally of significance with modern blood gas machines.

FiO$_2$

The fraction of the inspired breathing gas that is oxygen. In atmospheric air, the FiO$_2$ is ~ 0.21 (21%). When an anaesthetised patient is breathing a mixture of gases, which will be oxygen plus, for example, air and a volatile agent, the FiO$_2$ is that volume of oxygen (including the oxygen in the administered air) expressed as a fraction of the total gas flow. As a rough guide, pO$_2$ (arterial O$_2$ pressure) will be 10 kPa less than the % FiO$_2$ e.g., if FiO$_2$ is 50%, pO$_2$ will normally be 40 kPa. Administered FiO$_2$ is not usually greater than 0.5, otherwise the patient may suffer oxygen toxicity.

Fixed Acid

A **non-volatile** (not breathed out) **metabolic** acid (eg, ketones, lactate, phosphate, and sulphate), produced as a result of incomplete metabolism. All acids produced in the body, except carbonic acid (H_2CO_3) are fixed acids, and are removed by the kidneys.

Glucose

An important topic for monitoring, especially in diabetes mellitus patients, when insulin levels are too low to service glucose, or when glucose levels are too low, because that causes ketones to be formed, which can then lead to ketoacidosis.

Glycolysis

The process, and first part of cellular respiration, of producing pyruvate from the break down (by enzymes) of glucose: one glucose molecule converts to two molecules of pyruvic, two H+ ions, and two water molecules. In the presence of oxygen, pyruvate follows an aerobic pathway to be broken down for energy release. In a low oxygen situation, pyruvate is converted into lactate, to enable energy production.

H+

A positive hydrogen atom (cation), consisting of a proton only. H+ ions are what make acidity in the body, as measured by pH. The concentration of H+ ions is signified by square brackets: [H+].

Haematocrit (Hct)

Packed Cell Volume: Fraction of blood volume that is red blood cells. Reflects blood viscosity, and haemoglobin level. A low level causes

Appendix 1: Glossary

hypoxia. Normal range is 40 - 52% in men, and 36 - 48% in women.

Haemoglobin (Hb)

Complex protein molecule within red blood cells (~270 million/cell), which give them their colour, and by which CO_2 and 98% of oxygen is transported. The fraction of haemoglobin, which carries oxygen (oxyhaemoglobin), is the measurement for oxygen saturation. Normal range of arterial haemoglobin is 140 to 180 g/litre for men, and 120 to 160 g/litre for women. A low Hb count might be due to iron deficiency, anaemia, cancer, vitamin deficiency, hypothyroidism, pregnancy, urinary infection, liver disease, or low pH. Note: If Hb level is normal, but some of the Hb is defective (can't bind wth O_2), oxygen saturation (SO_2) will be low, but pO_2 may be normal, because pO_2 is measured in the plasma, not in Hb. See *Methaemoglobin, Carboxyhaemoglobin*.

Haemoglobin Electrophoresis

A system to determine what types of haemoglobin are contained within a blood sample, particularly useful when carbon monoxide (CO) poisoning is suspected, because CO binds to haemoglobin (Hb) in preference to oxygen, which means that even if the patient has a normal level of Hb, the CO will prevent some oxygen from binding to the Hb, and so the patient could become hypoxic.

HAGMA

See Appendix 8.

HCO_3^-

Chemical symbol for Bicarbonate. For simplicity, the minus sign (negatively charged ion) is often omitted in the text.

Hyperchloraemic Metabolic Acidosis

Acidotic condition caused by loss of bicarbonate (HCO_3^-), rather than an excess of acid (H^+). To maintain an electrical neutral state, Cl^- (chloride ions) shift from the cells and into the extracellular space, so causing an increase in serum Cl^-, and a more normal anion gap.

Seen in *Normal Anion Gap* metabolic acidosis.

Hyperkalaemia

Hyperkalaemia is an excess of potassium (> 5.2 mmol/litre), which the kidneys are unable to excrete, and may result in cardiac arrest. Causes include: Metabolic acidosis, endocrine problems, drugs, renal failure. Treatment is to give calcium or sodium bicarbonate. Note: *An acid condition causes potassium to move from cells into the plasma (to protect the heart), and $H+$ ions in the other direction.*

Hypernatraemia

Excess sodium in the blood (> 145 mmol/litre). Symptoms: *lethargy, tremors, irritability, seizures.* Treatment is governed by the underlying condition, and usually involves fluid based therapy.

Hyperventilation

Breathing too heavily, which can cause hypocapnia and respiratory alkalosis to develop. Commonly caused by anxiety, but also: fever, infection, drugs, pulmonary embolism, pregnancy, COPD. Can lead to exhaustion, which results in rapid increase in CO_2 retention.

Hypokalaemia

A serum potassium level of less than 3.5 mmol/litre, and which can cause arrhythmias, metabolic alkalosis, and cardiac arrest. Typically due to dehydration, laxatives, diuretics, steroids, drugs, vomiting, metabolic alkalosis, burns, kidney problems, low magnesium, hypothermia.

Hyponatraemia

A low blood serum sodium concentration which, according to N.I.C.E., is the most common electrolyte disorder. Common causes are diuretics and hypotonic fluids. Normal range: 136-142 mmol/litre; *Mild* hyponatraemia: 130-135; *Moderate*: 125-129; *Severe*: less than 125. Endocrinologist advice may be needed for all but the mildest cases.

Hypoventilation

Aka *respiratory depression*: Inadequate alveolar ventilation, resulting in increased CO_2 (carbon dioxide) concentration, and an increased acidic condition. Central chemoreceptors detect the high level of CO_2 (in the form of carbonic acid and H+ ions), and this triggers an increased respiratory drive, with the aim of flushing out the excess CO_2.

Hypoxaemia

Low partial pressure of oxygen in the blood. When breathing room air, a low partial pressure of oxygen (pO_2) in arterial blood is less than 10 kPa (75 mmHg), giving less than 90% saturation. If pO_2 drops below 8 kPa (60 mmHg), it is classed as Respiratory Failure Type I, unless the patient is also hypercapnic (high carbon dioxide), with pCO_2 > 6 kPa (45 mmHg), in which case it is Respiratory Failure Type II. Cells deprived of oxygen produce lactate, because absence of oxygen results in anaerobic metabolism. A common cause of hypoxaemia is V/Q mismatch.

Ion

An atom, molecule, or compound that does not have the same number of protons as electrons. Fewer electrons means the atom etc has an overall positive charge, and is termed a *cation*. Conversely, an extra electron produces an *anion*, and gives an overall negative charge. Removing an electron from a potassium (K) atom, for example, produces a cation, with symbol K+, as seen on blood gas reports.

Isotope

In addition to protons, the nucleus also contains neutrons, and the number of neutrons can differ between atoms of the same element type. For example, every carbon atom has 6 protons, but not the same number of neutrons. Some have 6 neutrons, some have 7, and others have 8. By adding the number of protons and neutrons, the version of that element is identified. For example, if a carbon atom contains 6 neutrons, that carbon atom is known as carbon-12, because it has 6 protons and 6 neutrons. Similarly, a carbon atom that has 7 neutrons is known as carbon-13, and so on. These different versions of the same element (atom) type are called "isotopes".

Think of it like a selection of cups of different types of coffee; they are all cups of coffee, but each has a very different and unique taste - a sort of selection of coffee isotopes (you get the drift). Any element that can have different numbers of neutrons will have its average (mean) number of electrons recorded on the Periodic Table. For example, the mean number of neutrons of all carbon atoms is 6.01 which, clearly, suggests that most carbon atoms are of the carbon-12 type.

K+

See Potassium.

Ketoacidosis

Ketone production that culminates in a metabolic acidosis. {Alcoholism can also cause ketoacidosis}

Ketones

A water soluble acidic compound produced when the liver breaks down fatty acids, measured in urine, which then enter the bloodstream for eventual use in energy production, during fasting periods, or when there is insufficient insulin for normal metabolism of glucose but, instead, fat and protein are broken down for energy.

Kidney Failure

Can cause decreased acid excretion, and increased bicarbonate excretion.

Lactate

A byproduct of anaerobic respiration (cells "producing" energy without oxygen), and often an indicator of sepsis, although modern thinking is questioning this perception. The liver is the primary organ for clearing lactate from the blood (converts to glucose), but the kidneys and muscles also make a contribution to clearance. Generally, and unless other information suggests otherwise, a high lactate level indicates a problem with oxygenation (**Type A** lactic acidosis), so referring to SO_2 and pO_2 must be part of the consideration of lactate level. High lactate might also be due to dehydration, liver or kidney failure, sepsis, hypoperfusion, hypoxaemia, or shock. Range: 0.5-2.2 mmol/litre.

Lactic Acidosis

A HAGMA acidosis, often due to anaerobic metabolism, that may be due to hypoxia, shock, or sepsis – a high white blood cell count can signify sepsis (from Full Blood Count). Lactic acidosis is where lactate is > 4 mmol/litre, and is of two types: **Type A** is is an excess of lactate as a consequence of hypoxia, as occurs with hypoperfusion in cardiac arrest, lung disease/oedema, hypovolaemia, or shock (haemorrhagic, obstructive, cardiogenic). **Type B** does not have a hypoxic cause, but is due to genetic and liver problems, burns, carbon monoxide poisoning, smoke, ketoacidosis, tumours, liver failure, low thiamine, organ ischaemia, or ingestion of toxic substances. Type B occurs in normal perfusion, oxygenation, blood pressure, blood volume, and normal Hb levels. Consequently, some septic patients can have lactate build-up even when oxygenation is normal.

Metabolic Acidosis

The condition where arterial pH is less than 7.4 (< 7.35 = acidaemia), unless compensated, and bicarbonate (HCO_3^-) ion level is less than 22 mmol/L (22 mEq/L). **Causes**: increased acid production or ingestion, serum bicarbonate loss, severe diarrhoea (loses bicarbonate), hypoventilation, organic acids (lactate, ketones), fasting, alcohol, toxins, inability of the kidneys to excrete excess acid, anaerobic metabolism. **Symptoms**: tachycardia, tachypnoea, fatigue, headache, nausea, loss of appetite, confusion, breathing difficulty, vomiting. Common **treatment** is to give sodium bicarbonate (if NAGMA) to buffer (mop up) H+ ions, and address the underlying cause.

Metabolic Acidosis: Respiratory Compensation

CO_2 compensation for metabolic acidosis is calculated by Winter's Formula: expected pCO_2 = (1.5 * HCO_3^-) + 8 mmHg (+/- 2). If pCO_2 is higher than calculated, it is evidence that a respiratory acidosis may also be present.

Appendix 1: Glossary

Metabolic Alkalosis

Raised pH, above 7.4 (> 7.45 is alkalaemia) due to either ① loss of H+ ions from vomiting or dehydration, or ② HCO_3^- (bicarbonate) retention, or HCO_3^- shifting into the cells. Underlying **causes**: diuretics, ingestion of alkali substances, severe vomiting (loses H+), bicarbonate infusion, severe dehydration, kidneys retaining bicarbonate. Usually accompanied by low potassium (K+) and chloride (Cl-) levels. Mixed metabolic and respiratory alkalosis might be due to liver cirrhosis.

Metabolic Alkalosis: Respiratory Compensation

An expected respiratory acidotic compensation (to normalise pH) with CO_2 is calculated as: $paCO_2 \sim (0.6 * \{HCO_3^- - 24\}) + 40$ mmHg (+/- 2). If blood gas $paCO_2$ is lower than expected, there may be a mixed respiratory/metabolic alkalosis. Conversely, a higher than expected blood gas level of $paCO_2$ suggests a mixed metabolic alkalosis/respiratory acidosis.

Metabolite

A substance produced when the body breaks down food, tissue, or chemicals.

Methaemoglobin (MetHb)

A form of haemoglobin that cannot carry oxygen.

Methaemoglobinaemia

Blood contains high levels of methaemoglobin. Treatments include hyperbaric oxygen and red blood cell transfusion.

Minute Volume
The product of respiratory rate and tidal volume.

Mole
Atoms and molecules are so small and numerous, that it is impossible to count and weigh them, so a reference value has been created from the carbon-12 isotope; a mole of carbon-12 atoms is the number of those atoms that produce a total mass of 12 g. That number (Avogadro's Number) is ~ 6.022 followed by 23 "0"s, or 600 billion trillion +.

Molecule
When two or more atoms of the same element bond (combine), they become a molecule. The oxygen we breathe, for example, is not individual oxygen atoms, but molecules of 2 atoms each, symbol O_2, known as molecular oxygen.

Na+
See Sodium.

NAGMA
See Appendix 8.

O₂Ct (Oxygen Content)
Total volume of oxygen dissolved in plasma and bound to haemoglobin:
$O_2Ct = (1.34 * Hb * SaO_2) + (0.003 * paO_2)$ ml.

O₂Hb
See Oxyhaemoglobin.

Appendix 1: Glossary

Oximetry

Measurement of oxygen and haemoglobin (Hb).

Oxygen-Haemoglobin Dissociation Curve

Describes how arterial oxygen saturation (SO$_2$) of Hb increases as arterial oxygen partial pressure (pO$_2$) increases, non-linearly.

Oxygenation Index

A calculation that can reveal lung problems, and illustrates how well the arteries have been oxygenated, for particular values of MAP (mean airway pressure), in cmH$_2$O, arterial oxygen partial pressure (mmHg, pO$_2$), and fraction (%) of inspired oxygen (FiO$_2$) * 100:

> FiO$_2$ * MAP * 100 / pO$_2$ or
>
> MAP * 100 * reciprocal of P/F Ratio

A high value, such as **10**, suggests poorer respiratory function, and a lower value, reflects better function.

Oxyhaemoglobin (O$_2$Hb)

A haemoglobin (Hb) molecule bound with oxygen molecules – to a maximum of four oxygen molecules per Hb.

PCO$_2$

Partial pressure of arterial carbon dioxide, with normal range being 4.7–6 kPa (35-45 mmHg). Hypoventilation causes a high level of CO$_2$, because minute volume is too low to blow off enough CO$_2$ to maintain a normal level, resulting in an acidic state, where pH is drops. Hyperventilation does the opposite, it blows off too much CO$_2$, resulting in an alkalotic (pH high) condition. Note: If an asthmatic patient is hypoxic and has a normal pCO2 level, it signifies deterioration and fatigue, and monitoring in a high dependency unit is necessary.

Periodic Table

The periodic table can be found in science books and many websites - it is very accessible. In the table, elements are arranged in ascending order of their atomic number – the number of protons in each element, starting with hydrogen, because it only has one proton. Information about each element includes its name, atomic number, name, symbol, and relative atomic mass, e.g.,

P/F Ratio

The ratio of the partial pressure of oxygen in the arteries, against the *Fraction of inspired Oxygen*: paO2/FiO2. An easy and useful measurement of pulmonary condition, and how well the patient's blood is being oxygenated from the alveoli and, hence, whether underlying causes, such as intra pulmonary shunt, might be present. For example, if paO2 is 105 mmHg, and FiO2 is 0.21, paO2/FiO2, 105/0.21 = 500. A value of 400-500 (at STP) is considered "normal"; anything lower than 300 might indicate hypoxaemia or lung damage.

pH

Potential or Power of Hydrogen: The value that describes how acid or base (alkali) an aqucous solution is, using a value between 0 and 14. The value is derived from the negative log10 of the H+ (hydrogen ion) concentration, in moles per litre of substance, and where the H+ concentration is signified as [H+]. Formally: pH = -log10 [H+].

At a pH of 7, the solution has equal concentrations of free hydrogen

Appendix 1: Glossary

(H+) and hydroxyl ions, of approximately 100 nanomoles per litre. If lower than 7, the solution is acidic and, above 7, the solution is alkali. For humans, normal pH range is 7.35-7.45; values outside this range prevent normal enzyme function, and can denature proteins, so maintaining acid-base balance is essential for health.

An ideal value of 7.4 means [H+] is ~40 nanomoles/litre. When pH is **low** (acidic), the kidneys (Loop of Henle) reabsorb bicarbonate (H+ buffer), and excrete H+. Additionally, low pH causes the serum potassium level to rise, because potassium moves from the cells and into the intravascular space. When pH is **high** (alkali), the kidneys remove more bicarbonate, but fewer H+ ions.

PCO_2

Partial pressure of carbon dioxide. Proper ventilation maintains arterial partial pressure of CO_2.

PO_2

The partial pressure of oxygen (O_2), dissolved in plasma (2% of all O_2), which should be approximately 10 kPa (75 mmHg) below the fraction of inspired oxygen (FiO_2). When breathing room (atmospheric) air, the "normal" arterial oxygen pressure (pO_2) lies in the range 10-13 kPa (75-100 mmHg). Needless to say, hypoxia should be corrected as soon as possible, with supplemental oxygen (if prescribed), and the underlying cause addressed, such as: supply problem, pathophysiology, CNS depression, low Hb or haematocrit etc.

Note that if there is a normal amount of Hb, but some of the Hb is defective and unavailable for oxygen binding, pO_2 might be normal, but SO_2 uncharacteristically low, in which case carbon monoxide might be

Appendix 1: Glossary

present. See also Respiratory Failure.

Potassium (K+)

The major intracellular + electrolyte (cation), maintains resting membrane potential, necessary for normal contraction of the myocardium. Potassium also helps nutrients cross into cells, and waste move the other way. Excess potassium (hyperkalaemia) and deficiency (hypokalaemia) can result in serious cardiac arrhythmias. A low level of hypokalaemia is often associated with metabolic alkalosis. Normal serum range is 3.5–5.2 mmol/litre.

Respiratory Acidosis

A pH less than 7.4 (< 7.35 = acidaemia), with pCO_2 greater than 6 kPa (45 mmHg). **Acute causes**: CO_2 retention due to hypoventilation, atelectasis, pneumothorax, anaesthetics, alcohol, asthma, toxins or CNS problems effecting respiratory drive (eg, resp infection), airway inflammation/obstruction, opiate induced respiratory depression, chest trauma. **Signs**: breathing difficulty, tachycardia, confusion, headaches. **Chronic causes**: typically COPD, pneumonia, obesity. Note: chronic respiratory acidosis may have few or no signs. **Treatment** is determined by the cause, and may include CPAP, intubation, increasing minute volume, bronchodilators, oxygen. Note: Chronic respiratory acidosis and metabolic compensation seem similar to mixed respiratory acidosis and metabolic alkalosis, so the mixed case may be identified by the patient vomiting. Mixed respiratory acidosis and respiratory alkalosis can not occur.

Respiratory Acidosis: Metabolic Compensation

In **acute** respiratory acidosis, the expected metabolic alkalotic compensation with HCO_3^- = *24 + [0.1 * (measured pCO_2 − 40 mmHg)]*

(+/- 2). If the HCO3- is lower than the calculated value, a metabolic acidosis may also be occurring. In a **chronic** condition (hours...days), HCO3- = 24 + *[0.4 * (measured pCO2 – 40 mmHg)]*.

<u>Note</u>: *In its early stages, buffering of H+ ions for respiratory acidosis is mostly by phosphates and haemoglobin, before bicarbonate levels have built up to an effective level for significant buffering.* See Appendix 5.

Respiratory Alkalosis

A pH greater than 7.4 (> 7.45 is alkalaemia), with a pCO2 less than 4.7 kPa (35 mmHg). Sedation or reducing minute volume may lower pH to a more normal value. **Causes** include hyperventilation, fever, sepsis, asthma, pregnancy, stroke, myocardial infarction, pain, pulmonary embolism, meningitis, doxapram, liver failure. Can produce myasthenia gravis, CNS depression. **Signs**: blurred vision, palpitations, sweating, dry mucous membranes. <u>Note</u>: Respiratory acidosis and respiratory alkalosis cannot occur together.

Respiratory Alkalosis: Metabolic Compensation

In **acute** respiratory alkalosis, the expected metabolic acidic compensation of reduced HCO3- is *24 – [0.2 * (40 - measured pCO2 mmHg)]* (+/- 2). If the HCO3- is higher than the calculated value, a metabolic alkalosis may also be present. In a **chronic** condition, the formula is *24 – [0.5 * (40 - measured pCO2 mmHg)]*. See Appendix 5.

Respiratory Failure (RF)

A cardiac or respiratory dysfunction, where the lungs are unable to remove enough CO2, or supply sufficient oxygen to the systemic circulation, resulting in hypoxaemia, and inability to maintain proper metabolism, when breathing normal ambient air, at Standard Temperature and Pressure. Diagnosed by arterial blood gas and spirometry. Type I: V/Q mismatch and hypoxaemia, pO2 < 8 kPa.

Type II: Hypoxaemia and hypercapnia, pCO2 > 6 kPa (45 mmHg).

RF can be due to obstruction, COPD, obesity, trauma, opiate induced respiratory depression, poor compliance, inflammation, oxygen supply problem, bronchospasm, or pulmonary oedema.

Room Air

A term which has no precise definition, because partial pressure of oxygen in "room air" depends on what the ambient air pressure is, which changes according to altitude and temperature. Generally, just assume it means Standard Pressure (760 mmHg @ mean sea level and temperature of 0° C).

Salicylate Poisoning

Potentially lethal toxicity, most commonly caused by Aspirin overdose. Acid-base symptoms are a triple disturbance of HAGMA metabolic acidosis, metabolic alkalosis, and respiratory alkalosis.

Sepsis

A life threatening response to infection, which can cause multi organ failure, and rapid deterioration in the patient's condition, leading to death. Abnormal body temperature is a common indicator of sepsis, as is a high lactate level. Another indication of sepsis is a WBC (white blood cell) count that is either high, or very low. Generally, sepsis is associated with an acidosis, but alkalosis might also be seen in early sepsis. Unless oxygen levels are adequate to serve the extra oxygen needed in the poor perfusion occurring in the presence of septic shock,

Appendix 1: Glossary

peripheral tissues may switch to anaerobic metabolism, and lactic acidosis may develop.

SO_2

Arterial blood oxygen saturation level – the ratio of oxygenated Hb to deoxygenated Hb that is capable of carrying oxygen. For a normally healthy adult, acceptable values are between 95% and 100%, and 88% considered hypoxaemic. For patients with respiratory dysfunction, oxygen saturation may normally be lower; COPD patients, for example, may have "normal" SO_2 of 88-92%, so values have to be considered within the context of particular patients and cases. Users of blood gas machines should understand how their machine finds the value for SO_2; is it derived using pO_2 and the corresponding saturation value on the oxygen-haemoglobin dissociation curve, or is it measured by taking into consideration presence of carbon monoxide (CO)? If it doesn't measure CO, and CO is present, the SO_2 value may be erroneous. Also consider anaemia – SO_2 may be 100% but, if Hb is low, oxygenation may be poor.

Sodium (Na+)

The main extracellular cation (positive ion) of sodium. The level of sodium, as with any other electrolyte, has a significance of its own: hypo/hyper -natraemia problems must be addressed, as per normal diagnostic and treatment protocols. However, when dealing with cases of metabolic acidosis, sodium levels (along with potassium, chloride, and HCO_3^-) help to reveal extra information about the causes and types of metabolic acidosis the patient is experiencing, using calculations for Anion Gap and Delta Ratio - knowledge of these things is not necessary for developing the ability to identify primary acid-base disturbances, but are essential for deeper understanding of the patient's condition.

Range: 133-146 mmol/litre.

Sodium Bicarbonate
An alkalising agent that can be given in cases where bicarbonate loss has occurred, causing a normal anion gap metabolic acidosis, and when pH is very low in cases of high anion gap metabolic acidosis.

Sodium Citrate
An alkalising agent that is used instead of sodium bicarbonate, particularly with patients having kidney failure.

STP (Standard Temperature and Pressure)
These reference values were defined so that scientific measurements could be made under identical conditions, thereby providing consistency with, for example, volumes and densities of specific gases, when made at mean sea level. In 1982, the International Union of Pure and Applied Chemistry defined Standard Pressure to be 1 bar, and Standard Temperature to be 0° C.

Uraemia
The kidneys are unable to excrete urea, resulting in urine polluting the bloodstream.

Ventilation
Processes of moving respiratory gases into and out of the lungs.

Ventilatory Failure
Inability to clear CO_2 from the lungs.

White Blood Cell (WBC) Count

WBCs fight infection, and a high WBC count is often associated with sepsis.

Winter's Formula

Calculation to predict the arterial carbon dioxide pressure (paCO2) that should occur if there has been a functional respiratory compensation for a metabolic acidosis:

pCO2 = (1.5 * HCO3⁻) + 8 +/- 2 mmHg.

∞ If the blood gas paCO2 corresponds with the calculated value, a **respiratory compensation** is occurring.

∞ If the paCO2 is higher than calculated, there may also be a **respiratory acidosis** (mixed acidosis) present.

∞ If the paCO2 is lower than the calculated value, there may be also be a **respiratory alkalosis** occurring.

Appendix 2: Arterial Blood Gas Assay

Appendix 2: Arterial Blood Gas Assay

Entry	Description	Range
pO_2	Oxygen partial pressure	10-13.3 kPa (75-100 mmHg)
SO_2	Oxygen saturation	95-100%
Hb	Haemoglobin count	130-180 (m) 115-165 (f) g/L
pH	Measure of acidity ($-\log_{10}$)	7.35-7.45
pCO_2	CO_2 partial pressure	4.7–6 kPa (35-45 mmHg)
HCO_3^-	Bicarbonate concentration	22-26 mmol/L
Base Excess	Positive: too much base. Negative: too much acid.	-2 to +2
Na^+	Sodium – cation	133-146 mmol/L
K^+	Potassium – cation	3.5-5.3 mmol/L
Cl^-	Chloride – anion	95-108 mmol/L
Lactate	Unmeasured anion (acidity)	0.5-2.2 mmol/L
Glucose	High/low? in DM patients	3.6-5.3 mmol/L

Appendix 3: Acid-Base Balance

pH	pCO₂	HCO₃⁻	Acid-base Status (rules)
↓	✓	↓	(1) Metabolic acidosis (CO₂ normal)
↓	↓	↓	(2) Metabolic acidosis + respiratory compensation occurring
↓	↑	✓	(3) Respiratory acidosis
↓	↑	↑	(4) Chronic respiratory acidosis + metabolic compensation occurring
↓	↑	↓	(5) Mixed resp/metabolic acidosis
↑	✓	↑	(6) Metabolic alkalosis (CO₂ normal)
↑	↑	↑	(7) Metabolic alkalosis + respiratory compensation occurring
↑	↓	✓	(8) Respiratory alkalosis
↑	↓	↓	(9) Respiratory alkalosis + metabolic compensation occurring
↑	↓	↑	(10) Mixed resp/metabolic alkalosis

Appendix 4: Mixed Acid-Base Conditions

	Metabolic Acidosis (HCO_3^- low ↓)	Metabolic Alkalosis (HCO_3^- ↑)
Respiratory Acidosis (CO_2 ↑)	pH ↓ E.g. cardiac arrest, multi-organ failure, opiates	E.g. lung disease, taking COPD with diuretics or vomiting, hypokalaemia, NG suctioning
Respiratory Alkalosis (CO_2 ↓)	Sepsis, renal failure and hyperventilates, aspirin overdose, liver disease	pH ↑ Diuretic use in liver cirrhosis, diuretics, ketoacidosis+vomiting, NG suctioning

Appendix 5: Expected Compensation

Disturbance	Expected HCO_3^-, mmol/L (+/2)
Acute Respiratory Acidosis	$HCO_3^- = 0.1 * (PCO_2 - 40) + 24$
Chronic Respiratory Acidosis	$HCO_3^- = 0.4 * (PCO_2 - 40) + 24$
Acute Respiratory Alkalosis	$HCO_3^- = 24 - (0.2 * [40 - PCO_2])$
Chronic Respiratory Alkalosis	$HCO_3^- = 24 - (0.5 * [40 - PCO_2])$

Disturbance	Expected pCO_2, mmHg (+/2)
Metabolic Acidosis	$pCO_2 = (1.5 * HCO_3^-) + 8$
Metabolic Alkalosis	$pCO_2 = 0.6 * (HCO_3^- - 24) + 40$

Appendix 6: Oxygen-Hb Dissociation

SO_2	pO_2 (rounded)
97%	96 mmHg (12.7 kPa)
96%	86 mmHg (11.4 kPa)
95%	79 mmHg (10.5 kPa)
94%	73 mmHg (9.7 kPa)
93%	69 mmHg (9.1 kPa)
92%	65 mmHg (8.6 kPa)
91%	62 mmHg (8.2 kPa)
90%	60 mmHg (8 kPa)
89%	57 mmHg (7.6 kPa)
88%	55 mmHg (7.3 kPa)
87%	53 mmHg (7 kPa)
86%	52 mmHg (6.9 kPa)

Appendix 7: pH -> paCO2

pH	paCO2
7.1	70 mmHg (9.3 kPa)
7.2	60 mmHg (8 kPa)
7.3	50 mmHg (6.6 kPa)
7.35	45 mmHg (6 kPa)
7.4	**40 mmHg (5.3 kPa)**
7.45	35 mmHg (4.6 kPa)
7.5	30 mmHg (4 kPa)
7.6	20 mmHg (2.6 kPa)
7.7	10 mmHg (1.3 kPa)

Appendix 8: Anion Gap

Metabolic acidosis is an inbalance where there is more acid than base, and the Anion Gap (AG) uses this fact to confirm the cause of a metabolic acidosis, which can be High Anion Gap (HAGMA) or Non-Anion Gap (NAGMA), by deriving the number (concentration) of unmeasured anions, in mmol/L. Anion Gap is an indicator of the contribution that unmeasured anions (albumin, sulphates, phosphates, ketones, acetate, lactate) make to metabolic acidosis, using the calculated difference between the number of measured major cations and anions; *AG = sodium + potassium − chloride − bicarbonate*. (Because it has a low value, potassium is omitted from the equation)

The Anion Gap is affected by albumin levels so, in practice, the albumin level must be considered when analysing a blood gas, but is not necessary for the purposes of learning how to read blood gas reports, so its mention is excluded from this text.

Normal Anion Gap Metabolic Acidosis (NAGMA)

NAGMA is a hyperchloraemic metabolic acidosis − Anion Gap (12 mmol/L +/-4). NAGMA is caused by loss of bicarbonate (compensated by chloride), from either the GI tract (diarrhoea) or kidneys (renal tubular acidosis), or due to intravenous sodium chloride administration, which displaces bicarbonate. Other causes include Addisons Disease, acidifying salt ingestion, and pancreas problems. Alkalising treatment is normally sodium bicarbonate, or sodium citrate if kidney failure.

High Anion Gap Metabolic Acidosis

HAGMA is caused by a relative excess of unmeasured anions (organic acids), where a high level of those anions is most commonly caused by TRKL - Toxin ingestion (eg, aspirin), Renal failure, Ketones, Lactate. The high level starts at approximately 20 mmol/litre.

Giving sodium bicarbonate (or sodium citrate, potassium citrate) as an alkalising agent is not effective in HAGMA, because low bicarbonate is not the cause of the acidosis, but might be helpful in severe acidosis, when pH < 7.1, or in ketoacidosis, when pH < 6.9.

Books By John England

- **Glossary of Anaesthetics**
  http://amzn.eu/g4Ah8AO

- **Q & A: Anaesthetic Principles, Volume 1**
  http://amzn.eu/iIbr8eK

- **Q & A: Anaesthetic Principles, Volume 2**
  http://amzn.eu/4eKMyRe

- **Q & A: Anaesthetic Principles, Volume 3**
  http://www.amazon.co.uk/dp/B0876F7V6S

- **Q & A: Anaesthetic Principles, Volumes 1-3**
  https://www.amazon.co.uk/dp/B087BJ7YXW

- **Perioperative Topics: Test and Learn**
  http://amzn.eu/gMhiDvm

- **Q & A: Basic Life Support**
  http://amzn.eu/acoxDel

- **Science Glossary**

Books By John England

https://www.amazon.co.uk/dp/B08DMV7GM/ref

- 📖 **Pass Your Drug Calculation Test**
  http://amzn.eu/duk6uT7

- 📖 **Basic Drug Calculations**
  http://amzn.eu/d0SWt0c

- 📖 **Drug Calculation Workbook**
  http://amzn.eu/d39gtl3

- 📖 **Drug Calculation Examples**
  http://amzn.eu/76zGfkJ

- 📖 **Drug Calculations By Formula**
  http://amzn.eu/eW9SEg3

- 📖 **Advanced Drug Calculation Workbook**
  http://amzn.eu/7zDyFQh

- 📖 **Nurse Q & A: Anatomy and Physiology**
  http://amzn.eu/f6nRC6G

- 📖 **Q & A: Respiratory System**
  http://amzn.eu/7RqNNxa

Printed in Great Britain
by Amazon